Nuclear Medicine
in Clinical Pediatrics

Nuclear Medicine in Clinical Pediatrics

Edited by

Hirsch Handmaker, M.D.

Director, Nuclear Medicine
Children's Hospital of San Francisco

Jerold M. Lowenstein, M.D.

Chairman, Department of Nuclear Medicine
Pacific Medical Center, San Francisco

Published by THE SOCIETY OF NUCLEAR MEDICINE, INC., NEW YORK

Distributed by PUBLISHING SCIENCES GROUP, INC., ACTON, MASS.

This book is based on a symposium entitled "Nuclear Medicine in Pediatrics" held February 16–17, 1973. The meeting was cosponsored by Children's Hospital of San Francisco and Continuing Education in Health Sciences, University of California, San Francisco, Calif. Financial support was provided by Abbott Laboratories, Dunn Instruments, 3M Co., Mallinckrodt/Nuclear, Searle Radiographics, Picker/Nuclear, Radx Corp., Raytheon Co., and E. R. Squibb & Son, Inc.

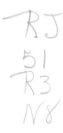

Distributed by
  Publishing Sciences Group, Inc.
  411 Massachusetts Avenue
  Acton, Massachusetts 01720

ISBN 0-88416-036-X

For Julius and Meyer Bloom, physicians,
for their inspiration, humanity,
and dedication to their patients.

Contributors

Naomi P. Alazraki, M.D.
Veterans Administration Hospital
La Jolla, California

William L. Ashburn, M.D.
University of California, San Diego
School of Medicine
San Diego, California

Edward G. Bell, M.D.
Crouse-Irving Memorial Hospital
Syracuse, New York

Willard J. Blankenship, M.D.
University of California at Davis
School of Medicine
Davis, California

Thomas F. Budinger, M.D.
Donner Laboratory
University of California
Berkeley, California

John A. Burdine, Jr., M.D.
Baylor College of Medicine
Houston, Texas

Richard Campeau, M.D.
Jackson Memorial Hospital
Miami, Florida

James J. Conway, M.D.
Children's Memorial Hospital
Chicago, Illinois

Gerald L. DeNardo, M.D.
University of California at Davis
School of Medicine
Davis, California

Sally J. DeNardo, M.D.
University of California at Davis
School of Medicine
Davis, California

R. Bruce Filmer, M.D.
Children's Memorial Hospital
Chicago, Illinois

Delbert A. Fisher, M.D.
Harbor General Hospital
Torrance, California

Gerald S. Freedman, M.D.
Yale University School of Medicine
New Haven, Connecticut

David L. Gilday, M.D.
Hospital for Sick Children
Toronto, Ontario, Canada

Hirsch Handmaker, M.D.
Children's Hospital of San Francisco
San Francisco, California

A. Everette James, Jr., M.D.
Johns Hopkins Medical Institutions
Baltimore, Maryland

Delores E. Johnson, M.D.
Harbor General Hospital
Torrance, California

Selna L. Kaplan, M.D.
University of California, San Francisco
San Francisco, California

James G. Kereiakes, Ph.D.
University of Cincinnati
College of Medicine
Cincinnati, Ohio

Joseph P. Kriss, M.D.
Stanford Medical Center
Stanford, California

Jerold M. Lowenstein, M.D.
Pacific Medical Center
San Francisco, California

David F. Mahon, M.D.
Upstate Medical Center
Syracuse, New York

Fred S. Mishkin, M.D.
Martin Luther King General Hospital
Los Angeles, California

Eugene T. Morita, M.D.
Mount Zion Hospital and Medical
  Center
San Francisco, California

William G. Myers, Ph.D., M.D.
Ohio State University
Columbus, Ohio

Victor Perez-Mendez, M.D.
University of California, San Francisco
San Francisco, California

Malcolm R. Powell, M.D.
San Francisco, California

David C. Price, M.D.
University of California, San Francisco
San Francisco, California

Curt Ries, M.D.
University of California, San Francisco
San Francisco, California

Eugene L. Saenger, M.D.
University of Cincinnati
College of Medicine
Cincinnati, Ohio

George B. Udvarhelyi, M.D.
Johns Hopkins Medical Institutions
Baltimore. Maryland

Contents

Preface

It is well accepted by the medical profession that pediatricians maintain a unique relationship with their patients and patients' families. This relationship begins at the dawn of life and frequently continues into adulthood, requiring the pediatrician to be neither first nor last to adopt new diagnostic and therapeutic methods. A realistic, cautious approach to the use of techniques involving complex technical information and equipment assures that the safety, reliability, and value of the studies is proven before they are made routine.

The rapid growth of pediatric radiology as a viable subspecialty is witness to this philosophy, and the use and contributions of the field are remarkable. In fact, there are pediatric "neuro"-radiologists and pediatric "cardio"-radiologists practicing in many centers. Caffey's desire for reduced pediatric patient exposure to ionizing radiation has been fulfilled by advances in technology and physician education (Caffey J, ed: *Pediatric X-Ray Diagnosis,* Chicago, Year Book Publishers, 1961, p vii). His concept of "minimal radiation dose" has a corollary later in this book (Chapter 16, p. 209). The similarities in the early beginnings of the field of pediatric radiology and pediatric nuclear medicine prompted us to solicit the comments of S. Scott Dunbar early in the preparation of this text because of his distinguished career in this field.

Equally dramatic to many of us in nuclear medicine has been the response of pediatricians to the applicability of nuclear medicine procedures to clinical pediatric problems. Again, because of technological advances (i.e., short-lived radiopharmaceuticals and improved detector systems) radiation exposures have become less of a deterrent to studying pediatric patients, and virtually all studies available can be performed in patients of all ages with "minimal irradiation dose".

The seeds for pediatric nuclear medicine were probably sown more than thirty years ago in Berkeley, as Myers points out in the Introduction to this book. Just ten years ago, a group of interested physicians met in Seattle under the auspices of Robert A. Aldrich, Professor of Pediatrics at the University of Washington, for the 45th Ross Conference on Pediatric Research, entitled "Clinical Use of Radioisotopes in Pediatrics". At that meeting a dozen topics were discussed, none of which involved the performance of an organ imaging technique. At the symposium held at Children's Hospital of San Francisco one decade later (upon which this text is based), 90% of the discussions dealt with such imaging procedures. It is no surprise then, that in this short time, transfer of the data from the nuclear medicine specialist to the pediatrician has been delayed.

In many instances, procedures have been revised and improved by the time the original work finds its way into the appropriate clinical literature. This publication is an attempt to deliver the latest and most pertinent information on the useful procedures avaliable to practicing pediatricians, house officers, and nuclear medicine specialists who only occasionally see pediatric patients. It is understood that even those of us devoting most of our time to pediatric problems may not be providing all we might in service. To this end, we have tried to provide a current and inexpensive source book to make available and better understood the relatively new techniques of "pediatric nuclear medicine". Speakers for the symposium and their collaborators for this publication are all recognized for their expertise in the areas they have prepared. Tables and appendices are offered as a guide to the specialist unfamiliar with pediatric doses, normal values, etc., but are just that—a guide—and reflect only the experience and opinions of the authors and contributors. We urge that all who use them recall that, as A. Graeme Mitchell quoted, "the child is not a little man".

All studies involving the administration of radioactive substances to children should be individualized to answer the specific question asked by the referring pediatrician and the appropriate material and dose selected. "Cookbook" studies should never become the standard of practice. We further urge the rational use of sedation to assure high-quality studies and to prevent reinjections. Our small patients and their devoted physicians require that we do no less.

We wish to express our thanks and appreciation to all those who worked hard to see this publication to its completion. For their constant encouragement and support, a special thanks to the Women's Board of Children's Hospital of San Francisco, and their President, Mrs. Charles F. Lowrey. For assistance in technical matters, thanks to Marye Rose, Rose Ann Anderson, Judy Fletcher, the staff at Continuing Education in Health Sciences, University of California, San Francisco, and all those at the Society of Nuclear Medicine.

HIRSCH HANDMAKER, M.D.
JEROLD M. LOWENSTEIN, M.D.

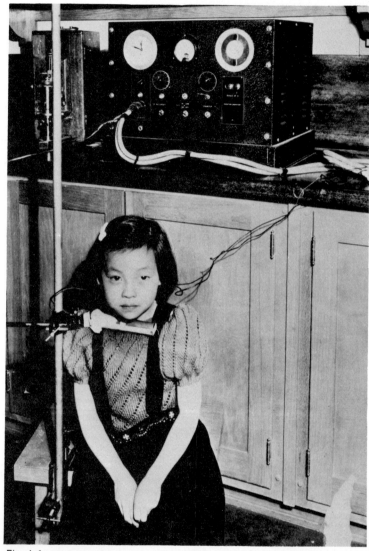

Fig. I-1. Method published in 1941–1942 (*1, 2*) for measuring the radioiodine uptake by the thyroid in situ by means of the interactions of penetrating γ-rays with a Geiger-Mueller tube placed against the neck over the gland.

Introduction:

HISTORICAL PERSPECTIVES

William G. Myers, Ph.D., M.D.*

> *Great institutions are but the*
> *lengthened shadows of great men*

Figure I-1 (frontispiece) depicts the method devised by Doctor Joseph Gilbert Hamilton (Fig. I-2) to measure the uptake of radioiodine by the thyroid gland in situ. The Geiger-Mueller tube was placed against the anterior neck over the child's thyroid. It detected penetrating γ-rays emitted from "inside-out" by radioiodine accumulating in the gland, as a function of time.

Figure I-1 was published first in a physics journal in June 1941 (*1*). Similarly, many of the early biomedical applications of man-made radio-isotopes first were described in physics journals. For example, much of the April 1941 issue of *The Journal of Applied Physics* contained brief disclosures of many varieties of such uses.

The picture in Fig. I-1 (frontispiece) was shown at a Symposium on the Cyclotron, held in San Francisco in December 1941. And it appears again in the November 1942 issue of *Radiology* (2). The seven papers presented at The Cyclotron Symposium fill this entire issue; and they constitute good sources of the early history of "nuclear" medicine during the first half dozen years after the announcement of the finding of artificial radioactivity in Paris early in 1934 (*3*).

It is appropriate, therefore, that the symposium on "Pediatric Nuclear Medicine" was held in San Francisco, just three decades after The Cyclotron Symposium there in 1941. For, the San Francisco Bay Area is the "cradle" of much of nuclear medicine. And many of the pioneers in this region are active still.

Here it was that Professor Ernest Lawrence and his coworkers (*4*) generated radioactive Nitrogen-13 in his cyclotron in Berkeley by bombarding carbon with deuterons, less than two weeks after this possibility had been projected by the discoverers of artificial radioactivity (*3*). Seven

---

* Historian of The Society of Nuclear Medicine. Professor in the Departments of Radiology, Physiology, and Medicine, The Ohio State University, University Hospital, 410 West 10th Avenue, Columbus, Ohio 43210; Visiting Professor of Nuclear Medicine, Donner Laboratory and Division of Medical Physics, Lawrence Berkeley Laboratory, University of California at Berkeley, Berkeley, California 94720.

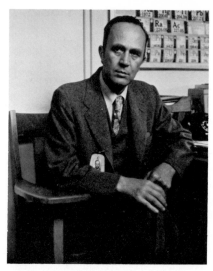

Fig. I-2. Joseph Gilbert Hamilton, M.D. He was the originator of "inside-out" assays in situ by means of γ-rays emitted by man-made radionuclides. He was born 11 November 1907 in Waverly, Massachusetts. This picture was made 23 April 1956 by the author at The Crocker Medical Cyclotron Laboratory (6) of which Doctor Hamilton then was director. He died of leukemia on 20 February 1957, in Children's Hospital in San Francisco.

months later, he became the father of nuclear biomedicine when he found that radioactive sodium could be produced with his cyclotron in multi-millicurie amounts and he prophesied (5) . . . "In the biological field radiosodium has interesting possibilities that hardly need be emphasized here" . . . When his 37 inch cyclotron went into operation in 1936 (7), it became evident that it was the only practicable instrument with which to generate radionuclides of "physiological" elements in amounts adequate for the zestful biomedical colleagues who soon clustered nearby to embrace new opportunities provided by the man-made tracer (9) "radio-indicators."

And among these workers was Ernest's physician brother, John Lawrence. After successful results in treating leukemic mice, Doctor John became the father of "radiopharmaceuticals" when, on Christmas Eve in 1936, he administered ^{32}P-phosphate to a patient who had leukemia (8). He and his colleagues published (10) their early findings with radiophosphate for treatment in more than 100 patients among the papers of The Cyclotron Symposium.

The 37-inch cyclotron was used in the discovery of two radionuclides that are used commonly in nuclear medicine today. Iodine-131 was announced by Livingood and Seaborg on 15 June 1938 (11). And, less than five months later, on 1 November 1938, Segrè and Seaborg reported on the discovery of what is now known as 6-hour Technetium-99m, together with the finding that it is the daughter of a 66-hour molybdenum radionuclide (*12*). It is estimated that more than ten percent of patients hospitalized in the United States now receive injections of a form of Tc-99m in various diagnostic procedures (*13*), chiefly when used in conjunction with a scintillation camera.

The next year, in 1939, Ernest Lawrence announced . . . "The medical cyclotron of the William H. Crocker Radiation Laboratory" . . . and that . . . "the yield of radioactive iodine is 20 times greater at the higher voltage" . . . generated by the new 60-inch apparatus (*6*). Later in 1939 he was awarded The Nobel Prize in Physics, and became the first of a dozen Nobel Laureates to grace the campus of The University of California at Berkeley, including Professor Seaborg (1951) and Professor Segrè (1959).

The impact of the successively enlarged cyclotrons on biomedicine was described ably by Doctor Paul C. Aebersold in his first paper of the 1941 Cyclotron Symposium on (*7*) "The Cyclotron: A Nuclear Transformer" and later (*8*) in his succinctly comprehensive survey of "The Development of Nuclear Medicine."

Presumably it was Professor Robert Newell at Stanford University who coined the name "Nuclear" Medicine (*14*). Because he anticipated many of the ramifications of this emerging new lore, he staunchly supported The Society of Nuclear Medicine in its early formative years. Also he gave us the focused collimator.

Professor Robert Hofstadter, also at Stanford University, discovered the thallium-activated sodium iodide crystal used in virtually all of the present scintillation detectors that are central to much of nuclear medicine, and without which inside-out imaging would not have evolved to its present state.

Hal Anger invented the scintillation camera in 1957 (*15, 16*) at The Donner Laboratory of Medical Physics, The Lawrence Berkeley Laboratory, on the campus of The University of California at Berkeley. And he displayed the first working model of this camera at the meeting of The American Medical Association in San Francisco in June 1958. The NaI(T1) crystal, which was only four inches in diameter and one-fourth inch thick, was viewed by seven multiplier phototubes. He demonstrated good images of the distribution of Iodine-131 in normal and diseased thyroid glands made with the pinhole version of this first scintillation camera.

By 1961, Anger's scintillation camera at The Donner Laboratory was equipped with a NaI(T1) crystal eight inches in diameter and one-fourth inch thick, which was viewed by nineteen phototubes. The first industrially-fabricated version of the scintillation camera, at this stage of development, was installed in the author's laboratory at The Ohio State University in September 1962 (*17, 18*).

A year later, Anger had built a scintillation camera with the diameter of the crystal increased to $11\frac{1}{2}$ inches and the thickness to one-half inch

(*16*). Since then, the thousands of scintillation cameras installed in laboratories throughout much of the world are used to make many millions of images annually; and . . . "The Anger scintillation camera has revolutionized the practice of clinical nuclear medicine" (*19*).

Anger has provided a scintillation camera at The Donner Laboratory for several years that is equipped with a NaI(T1) crystal sixteen inches in diameter and one-half inch thick which is viewed by 37 multiplier phototubes. Thus, it would be well suited for the making of "whole-body" images of distributions of γ-nuclides in small babies.

The I-131 (*11*) used by Hamilton and Soley in 1939–1940 (*20, 21*) was generated in Professor Ernest Lawrence's 60-inch medical cyclotron (*6*). The bombarded target contained natural tellurium, which is comprised of eight stable nuclides. Because indiscriminative Geiger-Mueller tubes were used for the inside-out assays depicted in Fig. I-1 (frontispiece), it seems probable that, when counting was done soon after bombardment, two radionuclides may have been involved (*24, 28*) which had not been discovered yet, viz. Iodine-123 and Iodine-125!

Professor I. Perlman used the same medical cyclotron (*6*) a decade later in the discovery of the 13-hour Iodine-123 (*22*), when antimony was bombarded with He-4 ions. Efforts designed to match the advantageous physical properties of Iodine-123 (13-hour half-life, 159-keV γ-ray, no beta particles) with the developing scintillation camera were reported briefly in 1962 (*23*). Especially significant for pediatric nuclear medicine is the greatly reduced radiation exposure, together with the much improved resolution of images, when cyclotron-generated I-123 replaces I-131 (*25–28*).

These spin-offs of Professor Ernest Lawrence's intuition now are recognized by the nuclear medicine practitioners and pediatricians who are embracing the commercial availability of I-123. This is because it is the "ideal" among the 29 radionuclides of iodine (*25*) for studies involving radiation exposures not exceeding a few percent of those from I-131, as well as for generating images having superior resolution by means of The Anger Scintillation Camera (*27–28*).

References

1. Hamilton JG: Applications of radioactive tracers to biology and medicine. *J Applied Physics* 12: 440–460, June 1941

2. Hamilton JG: The use of radioactive tracers in biology and medicine. *Radiology* 39: 541–572, November 1942

3. Joliot F, Curie I: Artificial production of a new kind of radio-element. *Nature* 133: 201–202, 10 February 1934

4. Henderson MC, Livingston MS, Lawrence EO: Artificial radioactivity produced by deuton bombardment. *Phys Rev* 45: 428–429, 15 March 1934

5. Lawrence EO: Radioactive sodium produced by deuton bombardment. *Physical Review* 46: 746, 15 October 1934

6. Lawrence EO: The medical cyclotron of the William H. Crocker Radiation Laboratory. *Science* 90: 407–408, 3 November 1939

7. Aebersold PC: The cyclotron: a nuclear transformer. *Radiology* 39: 513–540, November 1942

8. Aebersold PC: The development of nuclear medicine. *Am J Roentgenol Radium Ther Nucl Med* 75: 1027–1039, 1956

9. Hevesy GC: *Radioactive Indicators.* New York, Interscience, 1948 556 pages

10. Low-Beer BVA, Lawrence JH, Stone RS: The therapeutic use of artifically produced radioactive substances. *Radiology* 39: 573–597, November 1942

11. Livingood JJ, Seaborg GT: Radioactive iodine isotopes. *Phys Rev* 53: 1015, 15 June 1938

12. Segrè E, Seaborg GT: Nuclear isomerism in element 43. *Phys Rev* 54: 772, 1 November 1938

13. Wagner HN Jr: Personal communication, 19 April 1973

14. Brucer M: Personal communication, 11 November 1973

15. Anger HO: Scintillation camera. *Rev Sci Instr* 29: 27–33, 1958

16. Anger HO: Gamma-ray and positron scintillation camera. *Nucleonics* 21: No 10, 56–59, 1963

17. Myers WG: Scintillation camera for in vivo studies of dynamic processes. *J Nucl Med* 4: 182, 1963

18. Myers WG: Dynamic studies with a gamma-ray scintillation camera. In *Medical Radioisotope Scanning,* Vienna, IAEA, 1964, vol I, pp 377–387

19. Powell MR: Clinical applications of the scintillation camera. In *Nuclear Medicine,* 2nd ed, Blahd WG, ed, New York, McGraw-Hill, 1971, chapter 19 pp 533–573

20. Hamilton JG, Soley MH: Studies in iodine metabolism by the use of a new radioactive isotope of iodine. *Am J Physiol* 127: 557–572, 1939

21. Hamilton JG, Soley MH: Studies in iodine metabolism of the thyroid gland in situ by the use of radio-iodine in normal subjects and in patients with various types of goiter. *Am J Physiol* 131: 135–143, 1940–1941

22. Marquez L, Perlman I: Neutron deficient isotopes of iodine. UCRL-555, 1949; *Phys Rev* 189–190, 1950

23. Myers WG, Anger HO: Radioiodine-123. *J Nucl Med* 3: 183, 1962

24. Myers WG: Comparisons of I^{131}, I^{125}, and I^{123} for in vivo and in vitro applications in diagnosis. VIIth Int Cong Internal Med, Munich, 1962. In *Transactions* 2, Stuttgart, Georg Thieme Verlag, 1963, pp 858–863

25. Myers WG: Radioisotopes of iodine. In *Radioactive Pharmaceuticals,* 651111, AEC Symposium Series 6 Springfield, Va, National Bureau of Standards, 1966, chapter 12 pp 217–243

26. Myers WG: Radioiodine-123 for scanning. *J Nucl Med* 7: 390–391, 1966

27. Myers WG, Anger HO, Lamb JF, Winchell HS: ^{123}I for applications in diagnosis. In *New Developments in Radiopharmaceuticals and Labelled Compounds,* Vienna, IAEA, 1973, vol 1, pp 249–256

28. Myers WG: Radioiodine-123 for medical research and diagnosis. In *Recent Advances in Nuclear Medicine,* Lawrence JH, ed, New York, Grune & Stratton, 1974, vol 4, chapter 3, pp 131–160

Chapter **1**

Central Nervous System: Brain

Fred S. Mishkin

The pediatrician who requests a brain imaging procedure with radionuclides must recognize the limitations of the technique as well as its virtues so that the study may provide truly valuable information in solving clinical problems. Brain imaging (scintigraphy) can reliably solve certain problems such as excluding brain tumors, detecting over 80% of supratentorial neoplasms, and detecting 70% of infratentorial neoplasms. In some situations, such as cerebral abscess, the sensitivity of the scintigraphic technique rivals or exceeds that of more complex angiographic procedures. Other conditions, such as pontine gliomas, will usually show no scintigraphic abnormality in spite of clear-cut clinical evidence of the lesion. In view of this, it is difficult to maintain that brain imaging with radionuclides should be a "screening procedure" in pediatrics (1).

Performing Brain Scintigraphy

The gamma scintillation camera has made possible the visual estimation of the cerebral transit time of an intravenously injected radionuclide bolus. These studies should be performed routinely with all brain imaging studies on the assumption that one does not know with certainty before the study what pathologic process may be causing the problem. If the cause is known, then there is little justification for performing the study. Not only does the transit time study increase the sensitivity and specificity of the radionuclide brain image, but it also serves as a guide to the appropriate time for imaging after equilibrium of the radiopharmaceutical. Most lesions which cause abnormal radionuclide accumulation in the brain are seen best after a delay following injection. For example, many metastatic neoplasms, some primary neoplasms, infarcted regions, and subdural hematomas are best seen 3–4 hr after the intravenous injection of ^{99m}Tc-pertechnetate. On the other hand, some very vascular neoplasms, and some lesions which are seen primarily because of an increased blood pool such as arteriovenous malformations, may be seen very well or even best on early images. The great majority of such lesions appear as a blush of activity during the transit images (Figs. 1-1 and 1-2).

To avoid repeating studies unnecessarily and to reduce the risk of missing abnormalities best seen after a delay, imaging is routinely performed 3 hr after injection unless an area of increased vascularity is detected on the transit study. In this case static images are performed immediately (Fig. 1-3). Unpublished observations by Powell and Hand-

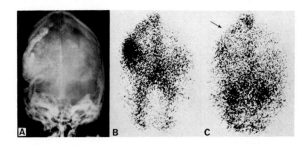

Fig. 1-1. Arteriovenous malformation shows more intense blush during arterial phase of flow study (B) than venous phase (C). Large draining vein (arrow) can be seen promptly filling sagittal sinus during arterial phase.

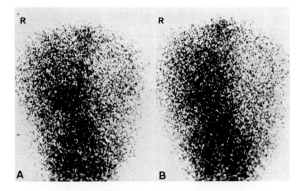

Fig. 1-2. Radionuclide angiogram in patient with hemispheric ependymoma shows blush in affected right hemisphere during arterial phase (A) which builds up during venous phase (B). Static images are seen in Fig. 1-3.

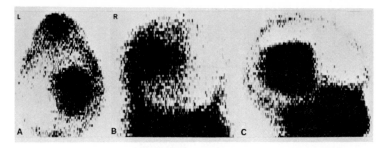

Fig. 1-3. Static images including vertex (A), anterior (B), and right lateral (C) views of highly vascular ependymoma were made immediately after flow study in Fig. 1-2 with no necessity for delay period for equilibration.

maker suggest that when ^{99m}Tc-DTPA is used for brain imaging the delayed image may be obtained as soon as 45–60 min after the initial injection without adversely affecting lesion detectability. Evaluation of a child's ability to cooperate is made at the time of injection. No hesitation should be made to sedate the child appropriately for the static images if he proves to be uncooperative (Appendix, Table A-1).

The routine static images should include anterior, posterior, both lateral, and vertex views. The vertex view proves extremely useful in evaluating problems of asymmetry which are common in childhood. Most of the activity seen outlining the head on the delayed image lies in the scalp and soft tissues of the head with the skull and brain normally contributing very little to the image. The dural sinuses serve as useful landmarks, particularly on the posterior view. To ensure that there is adequate flexion to allow imaging in the posterior fossa, the transverse sinuses should be projected in the midportion of the head in the posterior view.

The dose of radiopharmaceutical must be adjusted to the individual patient, but in general the recommendation in Table A-4A of the Appendix should be followed. Unless otherwise specified, all studies in this chapter were done with ^{99m}Tc-pertechnetate.

Clinical Indications for the Brain Scan

The problem responsible for referral of the largest group of children for brain imaging is *seizure*. Brain imaging is singularly unproductive in providing an answer to this problem, however. This is true particularly in the absence of focal neurological deficits (2).

Occasionally seizures themselves may, if prolonged, cause an abnormal brain scan (3). Laminar cortical necrosis may occur in the setting of a well-balanced, normal intracranial circulation. Deprivation of a critical nutrient (usually oxygen and occasionally glucose) for a limited period of time, or marked increase in metabolic activity (such as occurs with continual seizures with increased temperature) results in selective necrosis of the most sensitive cellular elements in the fourth cortical layer. This

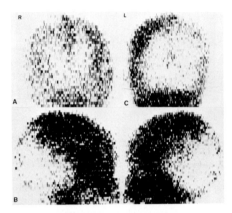

Fig. 1-4. Nine-month-old child had prolonged seizures with 40°C temperature and hemophilus influenza type B meningitis. Cerebral cortex was necrotic. No membranes were present. Anterior (A), posterior (C), right lateral (B), and left lateral (D) views mimic subdural hematoma.

abnormality appears as a mantle of abnormal activity over the brain and may mimic a subdural hematoma (Fig. 1-4).

Another common problem encountered in the child is that of a large head. In *hydrocephalus* the brain scan offers little more information than the cranial-facial disproportion apparent on the plain skull film (Fig. 1-5).

In obstructive hydrocephalus the supratentorial area enlarges at the expense of the infratentorial area with a relatively low position of the lateral sinuses which cannot be projected high on the posterior view, even with good flexion. Often the hydrocephalus is asymmetric. Occasionally the brain image may be more helpful as in the case of the *Dandy-Walker cyst.* This complex of anomalies, including cystic expansion of the fourth ventricle, agenesis of the cerebellar vermis, commonly accompanied by atresia of the foramina of Luschka and Magendie, occurs during

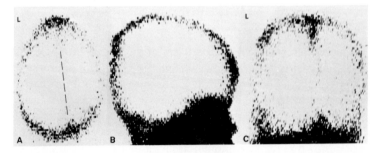

Fig. 1-5. Asymmetric hydrocephalus is seen best on vertex view (A) in which dashed line indicates course of sagittal sinus. There is increased activity in frontal bone seen on lateral view (B), probably related to increased skull growth in response to surgical decompression of hydrocephalus. In spite of good flexion of head, low position of lateral sinuses prevents their visualization on posterior view (C).

early embryological development when the lateral sinuses are in their primitive high position. Scintigraphy shows the high position of the lateral sinuses as well as the more acute angle made by the lateral sinuses at the torcular. Conway and his coworkers have pointed out that this angle normally averages 162 deg whereas in the Dandy-Walker malformation it is reduced to approximately 110 deg (4). Unfortunately, this is a nonspecific finding seen in a variety of cystic expansions in the posterior fossa such as a cystic cisterna magna and accompanying agenesis of the corpus callosum (Fig. 1-6).

Intracranial cysts may result in abnormal skull growth and deformity of the brain. Arachnoid cysts occur in a split in the arachnoid, expand and thin the overlying skull, and compress underlying cerebral tissue. They act as mass lesions, very similar to subdural hematomas or hygromas. In contrast, porencephalic cysts are atrophic processes usually lined with ependyma and communicating with the subarachnoid or ventricular space. Often the skull is thickened over such an atrophic area, but

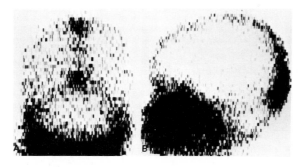

Fig. 1-6. Enlargement of posterior fossa without demonstrable cause. Angle of lateral sinuses can be seen to be more acute than usual on posterior view (A), and superimposition of sharply angled sinuses near torcular makes area appear quite dense on lateral view (B).

occasionally it is thin. It is important to detect large hemicranial arachnoid cysts since surgical resection may prove extremely beneficial to the child. Such cysts appear avascular on a transit study and may grossly displace the normal vascular pattern. On the delayed images the major dural sinuses can be seen displaced away from the abnormal hemisphere which is often expanded. The cyst itself, if large enough, appears on the delayed image as an area devoid of even background activity. Correlation with the skull roentgenogram may provide the final piece of evidence since a subtle degree of calvarial thinning is often present (Fig. 1-7).

Other congenital anomalies readily delineated clinically which have a high incidence of cerebral involvement may be fruitfully examined by the scanning technique. The *Sturge-Weber syndrome* is an example of such an anomaly in which seizures and a cutaneous angioma in the dis-

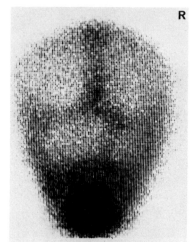

Fig. 1-7. Huge left cerebellar cyst enlarges left posterior fossa deviating midline activity to right and results in diminished activity. Asymmetric hydrocephalus with marked dilatation of left lateral ventricle accounts for hemispheric asymmetry.

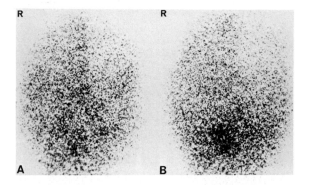

Fig. 1-8. Radionuclide angiogram in 13-year-old boy with Sturge-Weber syndrome shows increased activity of affected right hemisphere during both arterial (A) and venous phases (B).

tribution of the fifth cranial nerve or one of its branches are associated with an ipsilateral leptomeningeal angiomatous malformation. Underlying the anomaly there may be obliteration of the superficial cerebral veins so that venous drainage of the affected hemisphere is through abnormally enlarged veins, draining into the deep cerebral veins rather than over the cerebral convexity to the sagittal sinus. The radionuclide angiogram has a counterpart to the brain stain seen on contrast angiography with increased activity of the affected hemisphere seen particularly well during the venous phase (Fig. 1-8). Delayed images show that the affected hemisphere is smaller than its normal counterpart, with increased activity over the mantle of the hemisphere. This may be due in part to cerebral atrophy rather than directly due to the anomaly. One may also see abnormal uptake within the cerebral substance itself most pronounced in the occipital-parietal region where dystrophic cerebral changes and calcification occur most commonly (Fig. 1-9).

Arteriovenous malformations commonly underlie subarachnoid hemorrhages in children. The radionuclide angiogram can detect these malformations if they are large in size. Usually the arteriovenous malformation appears to diminish in activity from the arterial to venous phase of

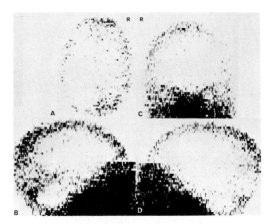

Fig. 1-9. Delayed images in Sturge-Weber syndrome show affected right hemisphere is smaller than left and has increased mantle of activity particularly well seen on vertex (A) and anterior (C) views. Increased accumulation of radionuclide can also be seen on right lateral view (B) in parietal-occipital area, region most often affected by dystrophic change and calcification. Left lateral view (D) is normal.

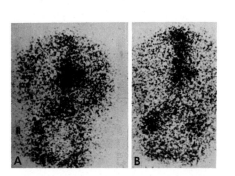
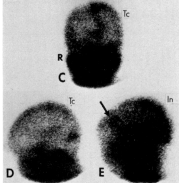

Fig. 1-10. Large arteriovenous malformation arising from anterior cerebral arteries can be well delineated on arterial (A) and venous (B) phases of flow study. Static images were immediately performed, showing lesion on anterior view (C) but not lateral (D) view with pertechnetate. Lateral image with ^{113m}In-chloride transferrin complex (E) shows lesion (arrow). Most of activity in indium image is in blood pools of major dural sinuses making it appear smaller than comparable pertechnetate image because scalp is not delineated.

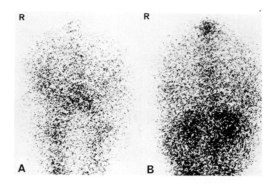

Fig. 1-11. Radionuclide angiogram in 11-year-old girl with occlusion of left middle cerebral artery shows diminished activity in ischemic left hemisphere during arterial phase (A) and increased activity during venous phase (B) due to late arrival through collateral routes and prolonged transit time of bolus.

the radionuclide angiogram. Abnormal early filling and enlargement of venous drainage of the anomaly may also be detected. In spite of early static imaging, it may be difficult to detect an arteriovenous malformation with an agent, such as pertechnetate, which is not retained in the blood. Immediate study with an agent which is retained in the blood pool, such as ^{113m}In- or ^{111}In-chloride, which binds to transferrin, or labeled albumin, may be helpful in difficult cases (Fig. 1-10) (5).

The sensitivity of brain imaging in detecting *cerebral ischemic disease* in childhood has been markedly increased by the addition of the radionuclide angiogram. In these patients the cerebral transit study will show reduced activity during the arterial phase and increased activity during the venous phase due to late arrival through collateral channels with prolonged transit time of the bolus (Fig. 1-11). The static images may show abnormal accumulation in the area of infarction, which in children

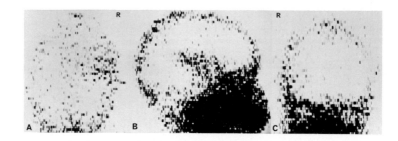

Fig. 1-12. Infarct due to right middle cerebral artery occlusion in 4-year-old boy is delineated by vertex (A), right lateral (B), and anterior (C) views corresponding with distribution of parietal branches of vessel.

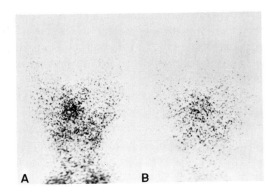

Fig. 1-13. Cerebral death in 14-month-old child maintained on respirator for 16 days is shown on flow study as absence of hemispheric perfusion on arterial phase (A) and venous phase (B). Injection is good as seen by visualization of carotid arteries in neck. Sagittal sinus is never seen.

almost always corresponds in location to the distribution of the major cerebral arteries (Fig. 1-12). A simple rule of three usually applies: that is, the delayed image is rarely positive within the first 3 days, is most positive in 3 weeks, and usually resolves 3 months after the acute clinical episode. There are, of course, exceptions to this generalization.

The most dire form of cerebral ischemia, namely, *cerebral death,* can reliably be detected by radionuclide angiography (6). The need to make this diagnosis hardly needs emphasis as once cerebral death has occurred further ventilatory assistance is futile. In cerebral death the appearance is unique. With a good bolus, the carotid vessels in the neck are well delineated and a hot nose signifying perfusion of the external carotid artery can be seen. Scalp activity can be delineated but no blush can be seen in the distribution of the major intracranial arteries and the sagittal sinus is not visualized (Fig. 1-13). This study can be performed very simply and

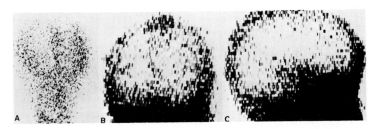

Fig. 1-14. Tuberculous meningitis has resulted in hydrocephalus causing splaying of middle cerebral arteries on flow study (A). Inflammatory process is most marked in interpeduncular area and results in abnormal activity in sellar region seen on anterior (B) and right lateral (C) views.

quickly with close cooperation of nursing and medical services for maintenance of respiration. While the single "flat" electroencephalogram has been questioned as diagnostic criteria for cerebral death, in combination with the radionuclide study pattern described, the findings may justify the diagnosis of cerebral death.

Children with *meningitis* are often referred for brain scintigraphy, but unless a chronic pachymeningitis or one of the complications of meningitis such as subdural effusion or cerebral abscess is present the scan will be normal. In *tuberculosis* the typical interpeduncular location of the proliferative pachymeningitis causes a characteristic scan abnormality which apparently is a poor prognostic sign (7) (Fig. 1-14). Ventriculitis associated with cerebral inflammatory disease and elevated cerebral spinal fluid protein can produce delineation of the ventricle (8).

Areas of *cerebritis* or *abscess* are detected with unrivaled sensitivity by the brain scan. There is evidence to suggest that brain scintigraphy will be the earliest abnormal study, suggesting a definite locus of inflammatory disease within the brain (9–12). Any child with a right-to-left intracardiac shunt who develops fever and headache should be a candidate for a brain scintigram to search for cerebritis or abscess. The scintigram will also serve as a convenient reference for following the results of therapy, whether medical or surgical (Fig. 1-15). Use of ^{67}Ga-citrate can be helpful in demonstrating inflammatory lesions which are

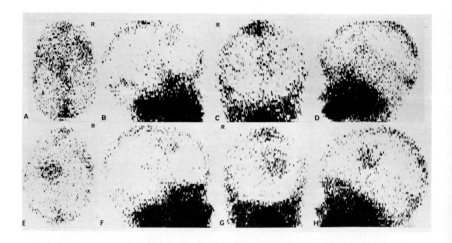

Fig. 1-15. Four year old with transposition of great vessels, ventricular septal defect, fever, and headache shows bilateral abnormalities on initial scan (upper row). Two weeks later (lower row), after systemic antibiotic therapy, lesion on right has regressed whereas lesion on left has becom more discrete and shows signs of central necrosis on scan below. Abscess required surgical drainage. Top row shows initial vertex (A), right lateral (B), anterior (C), and left lateral (D) images. E–H are corresponding images 2 weeks later.

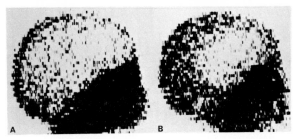

Fig. 1-16. Subdural hematoma. Right lateral view (A) performed ½ hr after intravenous injection of pertechnetate only suggests lesion which is well delineated on image 3 hr after injection (B). Patient was found to have subdural hematoma on arteriogram.

equivocal on the pertechnetate study. A variety of other inflammatory diseases of the brain including herpes simplex encephalitis have been reported, and scintigraphy will have an increasing role in the diagnosis of these diseases (*13, 14*).

Results in scintigraphic localization of *subdural hematomas* in children have, in general, been less successful than in adults. This may be due to a number of factors. A common problem with the use of pertechnetate is a failure to delay the image long enough after injection. At 3 hr the abnormality is much better delineated than after ½ hr. Often asymmetry on the frontal views is used as a diagnostic clue, but in children the subdural hematoma is often bilateral so the asymmetry is absent or not striking. In children the membrane of the subdural hematoma, which is at least in part responsible for the abnormal uptake, is poorly developed. Perhaps with increased use of routine delayed imaging, results will improve (Fig. 1-16).

Brain scintigraphy has been most widely used to detect *brain tumors,* one of the most common malignancies of children. Brain neoplasia tends to occur in peak incidence in the middle years of childhood. The radionuclide angiogram commonly shows a blush in the very vascular hemispheric neoplasms, primarily gliomas. The abnormal blush usually increases from arterial to venous phase and when present suggests the immediate performance of static images. Certain intracranial neoplasms of childhood present typical clinical syndromes (*15*). For example, large diencephalic gliomas may result in the diencephalic syndrome with extreme emaciation in spite of good appetite, hyperactivity, alert appearance, marked pallor, and a lack of neurologic deficit. The abnormal activity of these tumors merges with the activity at the base of the skull and because of this may be overlooked in spite of the large size (Fig. 1-17).

Tumors in the region of the optic chiasm and third ventricle are common in childhood resulting in visual difficulty and abnormal hypothalamic function. The majority of these may, if large enough, be de-

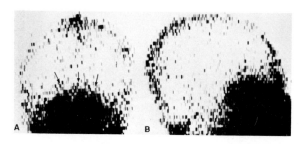

Fig. 1-17. Six month old with diencephalic syndrome due to huge undifferentiated glioma which can be seen bulging upward from base of skull on anterior (arrow) (A) and right lateral (B) views.

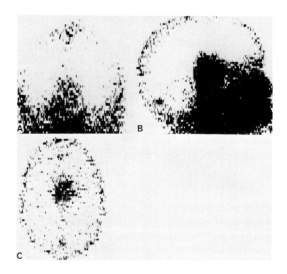

Fig. 1-18. Huge craniopharyngioma can be seen in typical location on anterior (A), right lateral (B), and vertex views (C).

tected by scanning technique. Craniopharyngiomas, which cause abnormalities on the skull roentgenogram more frequently than scan abnormalities in younger patients, may be detected on the scintigram (Fig. 1-18). The vertex view may be helpful in these patients (*16*).

Choroid plexus papillomas may lead to subarachnoid hemorrhage and hydrocephalus. These tumors may be detected using pertechnetate in spite of prior administration of perchlorate (Fig. 1-19). A recent report indicates that there may be some suppression of such lesions with administration of perchlorate but the authors fail to mention the time interval from injection to scanning (*17*). This may be avoided by the use of the ^{99m}Tc-DTPA chelate.

Pineal tumors may be detected by scintigraphy but may be difficult to distinguish from tumors in the cerebellar vermis lying at the free edge

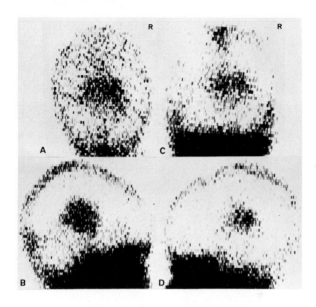

Fig. 1-19. Choroid plexus papilloma in four-year-old girl is well seen in spite of prior administration of perchlorate. A is vertex, C posterior, B right lateral, and D left lateral view.

of the tentorium. Reference to the skull roentgenograms may be helpful since the pinealoma may calcify. Furthermore, if one detects a lateral shift of the pineal, an infratentorial tumor is much less likely. Some pinealomas are the histologic equivalent of the seminoma, and these dysgerminomas have a propensity to seed down the subarachnoid space (Fig. 1-20).

It seems unnecessary to say that posterior fossa tumors cannot be detected unless the posterior fossa is clearly seen. This can be assured

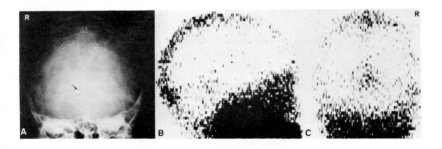

Fig. 1-20. Pineal dysgerminoma causes calcification and shift of pineal gland (A) but is barely delineated on right lateral (B) and posterior (C) views where it blends with dural sinus activity.

only if the lateral sinuses are projected in the midportion of the head on the posterior view. The slant-hole collimator for tomography with the gamma camera may prove useful for this purpose. There is no substitute for diligent supervision of the examination.

Medulloblastomas of the cerebellar vermis and ependymomas of the fourth ventricle tend to occur in the midline. On the posterior view they may be indistinguishable from a normal occipital sinus, and on the lateral view they occur low in the posterior fossa and merge with activity at the base of the skull. The patient with an ependymoma often presents with increased intracranial pressure without localizing neurologic signs whereas the patient with medulloblastoma presents with deficits in the vermis resulting in truncal ataxia and later develops increased intracranial pressure (Fig. 1-21). Cerebellar astrocytomas usually occur in the cerebellar hemisphere although they may be confined to the vermis or more often affect both the vermis and cerebellar hemisphere. In spite of the slow growth and cystic nature of these tumors they are almost uniformly detectable by the scintigraphic technique. Lateralization of abnormal ac-

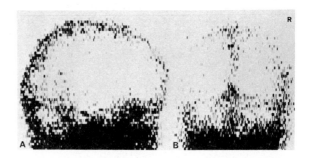

Fig. 1-21. An ependymoma occurs at base of posterior fossa as seen on right lateral view (A) and in midline on posterior view (B) where it mimics an occipital sinus.

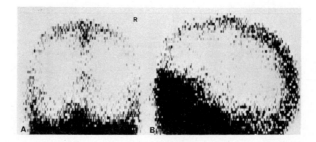

Fig. 1-22. Cerebellar astrocytoma accounts for abnormal activity in left posterior fossa on posterior scan (A) of 13-year-old girl who had varicella encephalitis 9 years before detection of tumor. Posterior fossa is filled in on left lateral view (B).

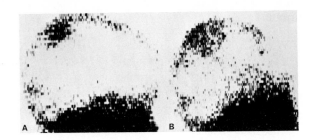

Fig. 1-23. Rapid growth of metastases from embryonal cell ovarian carcinoma can be seen over 1-month interval separating initial scan (A) from followup (B) right lateral views.

tivity occurs on the posterior view which tends to fill in the posterior fossa on the lateral view (Fig. 1-22). The child may present with limb ataxia without signs of increased intracranial pressure.

Pontine gliomas usually cause cranial nerve palsies before the development of increased intracranial pressure and show no brain scan abnormality with present techniques. An exception to this is extra-atrial extension of the tumor. This suggests that better technical means for delineating this region, such as tomography (*18*), may improve the rather miserable present results.

With increasing effectiveness of therapy for malignancy, secondary cerebral metastases are becoming more frequent. Radionuclide imaging provides a sensitive means for detection and a convenient method for following the effects of chemo- and radiotherapy (Fig. 1-23). At times the use of ^{67}Ga-citrate may prove helpful in defining lesions which are uncertain on the pertechnetate image.

Summary

Present radiopharmaceuticals and detector systems have provided nuclear medicine physicians and pediatricians with tools capable of detecting a variety of abnormalities with little radiation exposure. It is essential that the referring physician as well as the physician performing the procedure recognize both the limitations and virtues of these techniques. Appropriate selection of brain imaging procedures in each specific case must be the rule. Brain scintigraphy reliably solves certain problems, such as detecting or excluding intracranial tumors and identifying early cerebral inflammatory disease, cerebral ischemic disease, and a variety of congenital anomalies. Other situations, such as seizures without a focal neurologic deficit, acute meningitis, and hydrocephalus, are less often benefited by these studies. The role of these procedures in acute trauma and its sequelae is at the present time limited in pediatric practice.

Acknowledgment

Figures 1-1, 1-2, 1-7 to 1-9, 1-11 to 1-13, 1-15 to 1-17, 1-19, and 1-22 are reprinted from Ref. *1* with permission of Grune & Stratton. Figure 1-14 is reprinted from Ref. *7* with permission of *Radiology*.

References

1. MISHKIN FS: Brain scanning in children. *Semin Nucl Med* 2: 328–342, 1972

2. HURLEY PJ, WAGNER HN: Diagnostic value of brain scanning in children. *JAMA* 221: 877–881, 1972

3. PRENSKY AL, SWISHER CN, DeVIVO DC: Positive brain scans in children with idiopathic focal epileptic seizures. *Neurology* 23: 798–807, 1973

4. CONWAY JJ: Radionuclide imaging of the central nervous system in children. *Radiol Clin North Am* 10: 291–312, 1972

5. GENNA S, ZIMMERMAN S, PANG SC, et al: Four view dual nuclide imaging brain scintiscan analysis. *J Nucl Med* 14: 399, 1973

6. GOODMAN JM, MISHKIN FS, DYKEN M: Determination of brain death by isotope angiography. *JAMA* 209: 1869–1873, 1969

7. MAROON JC, JONES R, MISHKIN FS: Tuberculous meningitis diagnosed by brain scan. *Radiology* 104: 333–335, 1972

8. FULMER, LR, SFAKIANAKIS GN: Cerebral ventricle visualization during brain scanning with ⁹⁹ᵐTc-pertechnetate. *J Nucl Med* 15: 202–204, 1974

9. TEFFT M, MATSON DD, NEUHAUSER EBD: Brain abscess in children: radiologic methods for early detection. *Am J Roentgenol Radium Ther Nucl Med* 98: 675–688, 1966

10. DAVIS DO, POTCHEN EJ: Brain scanning and intracranial inflammatory disease. *Radiology* 95: 345–346, 1970

11. CAREY ME, CHOU SN, FRENCH LA: Experience with brain abscesses. *J Neurosurg* 36: 1–9, 1972

12. JORDAN CE, JAMES AE, HODGES FJ: Comparison of the cerebral angiogram and the brain radionuclide image in brain abscess. *Radiology* 104: 327–331, 1972

13. MISHKIN FS: Radionuclide angiogram and scan findings in a case of herpes simplex encephalitis. *J Nucl Med* 11: 608–609, 1970

14. HALPERN SE, SMITH CW, FICKEN V: ⁹⁹ᵐTc brain scanning in herpes virus type I encephalitis. *J Nucl Med* 11: 548–550, 1970

15. BELL WE, McCORMACK WF: Increased intracranial pressure in children. In *Major Problems in Clinical Pediatrics,* vol 8, Philadelphia, WB Saunders, 1972, pp 157–256

16. JAMES AE: Radionuclide imaging in the detection and differential diagnosis of cranio-pharyngiomas. *Am J Roentgenol Radium Ther Nucl Med* 109: 692–700, 1970

17. KAPLAN WD, McCOMB JG, STRAND RD, et al: Suppression of ⁹⁹ᵐTc-pertechnetate uptake in a choroid plexus papilloma. *Radiology* 109: 395–396, 1973

18. JAMES AE, LANGAN JK, FISHER CH, et al: Clinical experience in tomographic imaging with a tomocamera. In *Tomographic Imaging in Nuclear Medicine,* Freedman GS, ed, New York, Society of Nuclear Medicine, 1973 pp 206–219

Chapter **2**

Central Nervous System:
Cerebrospinal Fluid

A. Everette James, Jr., Richard Campeau, and
George B. Udvarhelyi

The gamma photon images obtained after placing an appropriate radio-pharmaceutical in the subarachnoid space have provided valuable information regarding cerebrospinal fluid (CSF) dynamics and are useful in the diagnosis of a variety of neurological abnormalities (1–6). Although anatomical detail is much greater with radiographic techniques, CSF imaging often provides a superior method of assessing CSF dynamics (7). The relative safety of the procedure compared with pneumoencephalography has made cisternography increasingly popular in neurological evaluation of children (3, 4, 8). A number of recent communications have discussed the use of CSF imaging in pediatric patients (1–6, 8, 9). From these it has become increasingly apparent that considerations of patient preparation, imaging times, pathophysiological mechanisms, and the clinical problems in children are sufficiently different from the adult population for "routine" studies used in older patients to be nonapplicable in many situations.

Patient Preparation

In our experience children between the ages of 6 months and 3 years generally require sedation. Infants less than 6 months can be immobilized without difficulty. Older children who understand the purpose and importance of the procedure may not require sedation. Restraints such as cloth sheets, taping, and binding boards should not be relied upon as the primary means of restraining an active child. The sedative mixture proposed by Conway (10) (Appendix, Table A-1) has proved reliable.

These doses should be decreased in very debilitated children and in those suffering from respiratory insufficiency. Vistaril may be substituted for Phenergan in children with seizures. The patient should be kept "NPO" for several hours before sedation to avoid possible aspiration of gastric contents. As a general guideline every nuclear medicine department performing pediatric studies should have pediatric resuscitative equipment immediately available for emergencies.

Since children, particularly young infants, have marked thyroid affinity for radioiodine (11), blocking of the patient's thyroid uptake should be performed in those patients receiving radioiodinated compounds. Three drops of Lugol's solution should be administered 1 day before the study and twice a day for 1 week after completion of the study. It should be noted that excess iodide may induce vomiting in young infants after several days (12).

Choice of Radiopharmaceuticals

A number of radiopharmaceuticals have been employed for CSF imaging (13). Consideration of anticipated length of study, pre-injection radiopharmaceutical testing, physical properties, and radionuclide availability are all important. Serum albumin labeled with ^{131}I (IHSA) has been most generally used, but because of its relatively poor photon yield and high energy of gamma and beta emission, we favor either ^{111}In- or ^{99m}Tc-labeled diethylenetriaminepentaacetic acid (DTPA), a chelate, or ^{99m}Tc-albumin (HSA). If the examination is to be completed in one day, ^{99m}Tc ($T_{1/2}$ 6 hr) is the radionuclide of choice. If delayed studies at 24–72 hr are anticipated, we would choose ^{111}In-DTPA ($T_{1/2}$ 2.8 days). Chelated radionuclides (MW 600–800) have been shown to have a movement pattern similar to labeled albumin (MW 69,000) (13) although somewhat less parasagittal concentration on later views is frequently observed (14).

Injection Techniques

The radiopharmaceutical is injected using standard lumbar puncture techniques. Ventricular and cisterna magna injections should be performed only by someone skilled in these methods. If percutaneous shunt reservoir injection is to be done in assessing shunt patency, strict aseptic

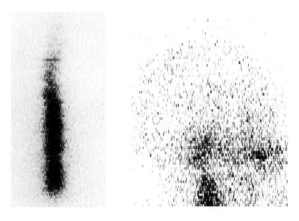

Fig. 2-1. (Left) View of lumbar spine 30 min after injection of radiopharmaceutical presumably into subarachnoid space.

Fig. 2-2. (Right) Right lateral skull view of cisternogram 1 hr after injection of chelate in extra-arachnoid space. Large amount of soft-tissue radioactivity as well as a concentration within extracellular space gives appearance of brain scan. There is radioactivity in cervical spine and basal cisterns, but anatomical detail is not sufficient for diagnosis.

technique should be used, in view of the significant morbidity associated with treatment of infected shunts.

Manometrics should probably be avoided during lumbar punctures to reduce the incidence of extra-arachnoid injections. We are not certain whether infusion tests should be obtained at the same time as the cisternographic images, but they will probably increase the percentage of improper injections. Improper radiopharmaceutical placement is a major problem in cisternography, occurring in 10–40% of reported cases. Recent lumbar punctures do not appear to have been predisposing factors to intrathecal injection failures. The patterns of significant subdural or epidural injections have been described recently by Larson and colleagues (15). In our experience, the epidural or "Christmas tree" and the subdural or "railroad track" patterns are much more common with radioalbumin than with the radiochelates. Figure 2-1 depicts what is seen commonly with an extra-arachnoid injection. The globular pattern is a reflection of the greater movement of the chelates (MW 600–800) in the extra-arachnoid spaces. Monitoring urine radioactivity in the first hour after injection will often detect faulty injections of radiochelates (16). Additionally, a 1-hr view of the cranium will have the appearance of a brain scan when extra-arachnoid placement of radiochelate (Fig. 2-2) has occurred.

Because faulty injections often involve deposition of radiopharmaceutical in the intrathecal space as well as extra-arachnoidally, the study

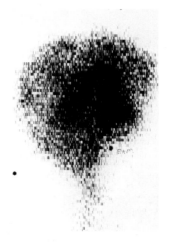

Fig. 2-3. Right lateral view of cisternogram at 6 hr shows large amount of soft-tissue radioactivity, but there is also enough anatomical detail to delineate lateral ventricular penetration. This is example of poor injection, but there is sufficient anatomical detail to give accurate diagnosis.

should not be abandoned at the time the clinician feels a faulty injection has occurred. Significant anatomical information may occasionally be obtained on later views, e.g., the presence of communicating hydrocephalus (Fig. 2-3). However, no attempt to assess the rate of absorption of CSF should be attempted if a faulty injection has been detected.

Imaging

Because of relative ease of patient positioning, scanning time factors, and facility in the quantification of radionuclide CSF clearance, we favor the stationary camera imaging devices in pediatric CSF imaging. In view of the more rapid movement of radiopharmaceuticals in children, imaging is best done at ½ hr, 1–2 hr, 6 hr, 24 hr, and longer if required to assess the clinical problem. In certain circumstances, such as shunt patency evaluation, imaging should be initiated immediately after injection. Figure 2-4 shows sequential images in a normal 8-year-old boy. Cisterna magna activity is noted on 30-min to 1-hr images. By the time of the 2-hr study, normal children should show activity in the basilar cisterns. At 2–6 hr activity will be seen to be ascending laterally along the Sylvian cisterns and medially through the interhemispheric cistern. By the 6-hr study the radionuclide will be present in the area of the cerebral convexities in 80% of normal children. At 24 hr the radiopharmaceutical should be virtually absent from the basal cisterns and present over the cerebral convexities or concentrated in the region of the parasagittal sinus. A point to be emphasized is that the radiopharmaceutical does not

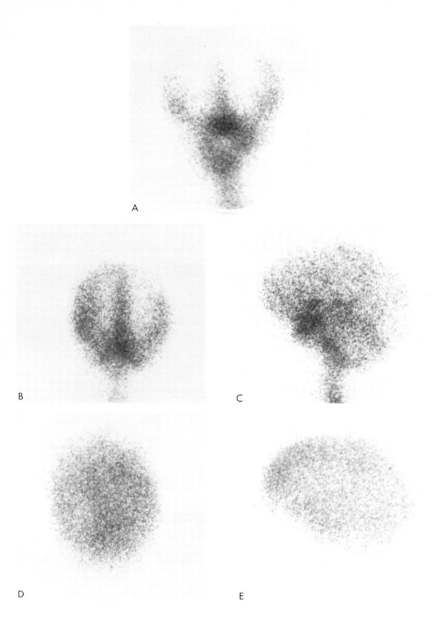

Fig. 2-4. Normal cisternogram obtained with ^{111}In-DTPA. (A) Anterior view at 2 hr shows radioactivity within basal cisterns as well as radioactivity beginning to move over cerebral convexities and in Sylvian cisterns. There is central radioactivity seen in linear fashion in sagittal or interhemispheric cistern. (B) Anterior and (C) left lateral cisternographic views at 6 hr shows further progression of movement of radioactivity up over cerebral cortex toward parasagittal region. There is still some basal radioactivity remaining which is expected. Most of movement of radioactivity is anteriorly and centrally. (D) Posterior and (E) left lateral views at 24 hr show homogenous distribution of radioactivity over cerebral cortex with some concentration in parasagittal region superiorly.

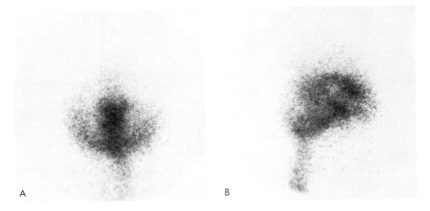

Fig. 2-5. (A) Anterior and (B) right lateral cisternogram at 2 hr demonstrate entry of radiopharmaceutical into lateral ventricles. This is characteristic sign seen with communicating hydrocephalus (9-year-old child; 500 µCi ¹¹¹In-DTPA).

normally enter the ventricular system. This is thought to be a reflection of bulk flow of CSF from areas of greatest production (choroid plexus of the lateral ventricles) to those of greatest resorption (arachnoid granulations in the parasagittal region).

Abnormal Radiopharmaceutical Movement

Figure 2-5 demonstrates a typical pattern of communicating hydrocephalus. This diagnosis can be made whenever ventricular entry of

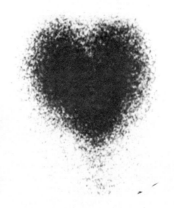

Fig. 2-6. Anterior view 2 hr after 500 µCi of ¹¹¹In-DTPA in 11-year-old child with extremely large ventricles. "Heart-shaped" collection of radiopharmaceutical is characteristic of that seen in anterior view of communicating hydrocephalus.

radionuclide is observed on the standard cisternogram (5). This entry is evidence that no obstruction exists between the outlets of the fourth ventricle and the cisterna magna. Medial radioactivity in the ambient, quadrigeminal, and interhemispheric cisterns must be distinguished from ventricular activity. With some experience this differentiation can be made in virtually all cases by examining multiple views. Figures 2-6, 2-7, and 2-8 show patterns of ventricular activity. In anterior (Fig. 2-6) and posterior (Fig. 2-7) views, ventricular radioactivity has a "heart" and "butterfly" appearance, respectively. In the lateral views (Fig. 2-8) ventricular activity has a "comma" or "C" configuration and should be distinguished from activity in the Sylvian fissures.

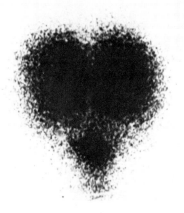

Fig. 2-7. Posterior view at 2 hr in patient with markedly dilated ventricles. This is so-called "butterfly" pattern seen on posterior view in communicating hydrocephalus.

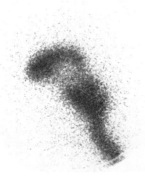

Fig. 2-8. Left lateral view at 2 hr in patient with moderately enlarged ventricles. "C" or comma-shaped area of radioactivity is configuration of communicating hydrocephalus formed by ventricular entry of radiopharmaceutical (500 μCi of ^{111}In-DTPA injected into lumbar subarachnoid space).

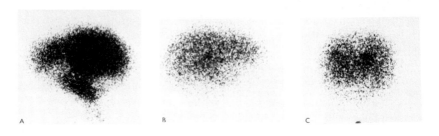

A   B   C

Fig. 2-9. (A) **Left lateral cisternogram at 2 hr in patient with markedly dilated ventricles which are well delineated.** (B) **Right lateral and** (C) **anterior views at 72 hr showing continued ventricular radioactivity which is characteristic of that seen with communicating hydrocephalus and stasis. Patient has markedly dilated ventricles with almost all of radioactivity confined to ventricular region on delayed views.**

In communicating hydrocephalus, two basic patterns are observed. In the first (Fig. 2-9), there is rapid ventricular entry seen on the early views (Fig. 2-9A). On later views (24–72+ hr; Fig. 2-9B and C) there is retention of ventricular activity with little or no ascension of tracer over the cerebral convexities. This pattern has been correlated with benefit from surgical CSF drainage procedures. In the second pattern of communicating hydrocephalus (Fig. 2-10) relatively rapid ventricular entry of the radionuclide is observed (Fig. 2-10A and B) but ventricular clearance is also rapid so that very little activity is seen in the ventricles at 24–36 hr (Fig. 2-10C and D). This suggests that partial compensation of the hydrocephalus exists at the time of imaging, and surgical treatment should be deferred. Careful followup must be obtained, however, since these children will occasionally decompensate. Quantitative cisternography (to be subsequently discussed) may be helpful in serially monitoring these patients.

It is probable that the pattern of ventricular stasis with dilated ventricles is simply the end stage of a process that often begins in the pediatric age group with obliteration of subarachnoid CSF pathways secondary to a previous meningitis or subarachnoid hemorrhage. These children recover from the initial episode but on serial cisternograms show progression from a pattern of delayed CSF movement, often with localized block, to ventricular dilatation with some "clearing", and finally to frank ventricular enlargement with marked "stasis".

In children with obstruction to flow within the ventricular system or at the outlets of the fourth ventricle (noncommunicating hydrocephalus), a normal cisternogram will be seen if the intracranial pressure is not elevated. With increased intracranial pressure the subarachnoid CSF pathways are partially obstructed, and one sees decreased movement of CSF with some degree of stasis in the basilar cisterns. Most often the diagnosis of noncommunicating hydrocephalus (Fig. 2-11) is made by ventriculography or pneumoencephalography. These children are very symptomatic and require immediate lowering of intraventricular pressure and subsequently a CSF diversionary procedure. If a ventriculocisternal shunt is contemplated, patency of the subarachnoid pathways into which the ventricular fluid will be placed must be assured. After the patient's ventricular pressure is lowered, a conventional cisternogram will be helpful in demonstrating the patency of CSF pathways from the basal cisterns to the parasagittal sinus.

In the evaluation of children with osseous spinal defects and meningomyeloceles, a CSF imaging study will often demonstrate an associated communicating hydrocephalus. If recurrent bouts of meningitis

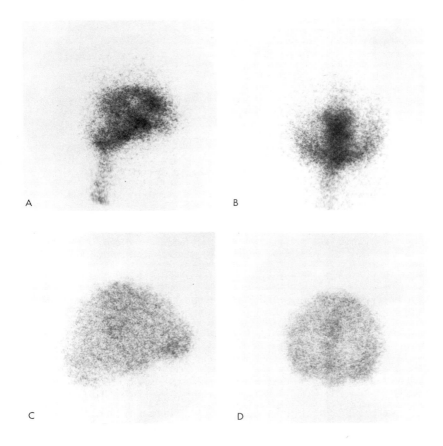

Fig. 2-10. (A) Right lateral and (B) anterior views at 2 hr of patient with communicating hydrocephalus. Ventricular entry is present. (C) Right lateral and (D) anterior views at 24 hr. There is clearing of radioactivity from ventricles and movement of radioactivity up over cerebral cortex with some concentration in parasagittal region. This is characteristic of cisternographic pattern seen with ventricular entry and "clearing".

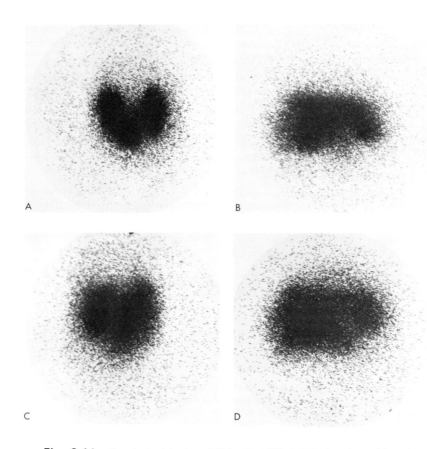

Fig. 2-11. Ventricular injection of 250 μ Ci of ¹¹¹In-DTPA. Anterior and lateral views at 20 min (A, B) and 72 hr (C, D) demonstrate continued radioactivity within ventricles demonstrating noncommunicating hydrocephalus.

are superimposed, inflammation may result in closure of the aqueduct of Sylvius and conversion to noncommunicating hydrocephalus. A problem that is particularly common in the pediatric age group is localized dilatation of the CSF space. Dandy-Walker cysts have been studied by both brain scans and cisternography. In general, closure of the foramina of Luschka and Magendie prevents entry of the radiopharmaceutical into the ventricular system from a lumbar subarachnoid injection. In patients with extracerebellar types of posterior fossa cysts there may be filling and even selective concentration of radiopharmaceutical within the cyst. Children with Arnold-Chiari malformation usually demonstrate a cessation of radiopharmaceutical flow within the cyst and at the level of the foramen magnum. Porencephalic cysts and subdural hygromas have been reported to selectively accumulate ¹³¹I-albumin (6). The retention of radiopharmaceutical may correlate with continued enlargement of these collections and serve as an indication for surgery. In our experience posterior fossa abnormalities are more common in children than in the adult population.

Pathophysiological Mechanisms

The CSF imaging pattern of ventricular entry and stasis in children with chronic communicating hydrocephalus has been well described and documented. The cause of this ventricular "penetration" and the reason the radiopharmaceutical remains there for prolonged time periods is not known. Radiopharmaceutical presence in the ventricular region soon after lumbar subarachnoid injection cannot be explained by molecular diffusion nor can it be accounted for by rapid transfer into blood and secretion by the choroid plexus.

To consider the possible explanations of these phenomena one must first recall the generally accepted relations of production and absorption of cerebrospinal fluid. The composition of CSF is such that it must be produced by an active process and does not represent an ultrafiltrate of blood. The site of greatest production is in the ventricular system. The choroid plexus seems mainly responsible although certain data support the concept that a significant contribution is from the ventricular ependyma.

Absorption of CSF in certain animal species is possible by the arachnoid villi of the spinal cord, the optic and otic tracts through lymphatic pathways and other unidentified sites. However, in the human and subhuman primate the major site of absorption appears to reside in the arachnoid villi in the parasagittal region.

Thus if the bulk of cerebrospinal fluid is formed in the ventricles and absorbed over the cerebral cortex, there is a resultant net flow of CSF out of the ventricles. This seems to be the most reasonable explanation for the radiopharmaceutical not entering the ventricles in normal children.

When the pathways of CSF flow between the ventricles and the arachnoid villi are either obstructed or obliterated, absorption of CSF is impaired. We have reconstructed this circumstance by using an experimental model for chronic communicating hydrocephalus. Initially, even though there is reduced absorption of CSF, production is not decreased. This relative overproduction causes an outward force upon the ventricles that (because it is a fluid-filled closed system) is reflected in increased pressure in the subarachnoid space surrounding the brain as well as the ventricles. Being a viscoelastic substance, the brain resists these forces but is somewhat compliant because of the presence of structures such as the cerebral veins (17). The cerebral veins may collapse, causing transient pressure necrosis. Following these pressure changes which occur primarily in the periventricular white matter, the ventricles enlarge, especially the lateral ventricles at their angles (Fig. 2-12). With ventricular enlargement the ependyma changes from the normal cuboidal pattern to a flattened one. In some areas the ventricular lining is denuded. With these histological changes the ventricular ependyma no longer acts as a partial barrier to CSF and its constituents. Cerebrospinal fluid and larger molecules (such as albumin) pass into the brain parenchyma, not by diffusion as in the normal but by facilitated diffusion (bulk flow). Quantitative autoradiography performed in our laboratory has documented these changes. As the ventricles enlarge so do the spaces between ependymal cells, facilitating this transependymal migration. This leads to an increase in the periventricular extracellular space.

After an unspecified period of time, ventricular enlargement may be offset by the increase in extracellular space, and further ventricular enlargement is resisted. However, this stable circumstance is achieved more slowly if the bony calvarium does not act as a permanent resistance to continued enlargement of intracranial structures, namely the ventricles. Thus before sutural closure, marked ventricular dilatation will be seen, often with only minimal neurological deficit. This is especially common in infants and young children.

With ventricular enlargement and transependymal migration of CSF the net flow out of the ventricle is lost. Since the ventricle may now participate in CSF absorption, the radiopharmaceutical enters the ventricles, passes across the ventricular ependyma, and remains in this enlarged CSF space for prolonged periods of time (stasis). It does not flow out over the cerebral cortex because CSF is not being preferentially absorbed there. These explanations are supported by gross and microscopic autoradiographs showing progressive penetration of labeled albumin in an animal with chronic communicating hydrocephalus. In children with ventricular "stasis" on delayed views, "apparent" ventricular enlargement occurs on the images probably reflecting transependymal migration in the clinical circumstance.

Shunt Patency Evaluation

Many new types of shunt systems are being designed, and there is constant reevaluation of the optimum combination of reservoir, valve system, and location of distal shunt placement. At present, ventriculoatrial shunts are most frequently used. Because of greater simplicity and less frequent surgical revision, peritoneal shunts are receiving renewed enthusiasm.

In general, radionuclide studies will accurately determine whether or not a shunt is patent (18, 19, 20). In patients shunted for noncom-

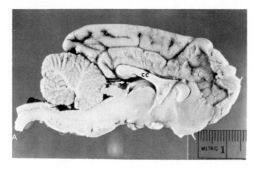

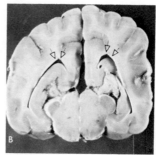

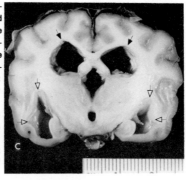

Fig. 2-12. Pathological specimens of animals after injection of silastic into subarachnoid space to effect block of CSF flow and produce communicating hydrocephalus. (A) Sagittal section showing minimal ventricular dilatation (white arrow), cc = corpus callosum. (B) Coronal section through lateral ventricles which shows that dilatation is beginning at ventricle and is mainly at expense of white matter (arrows). (C) Specimen in animal 45 days after silastic implantation demonstrating further dilatation of ventricles involving lateral ventricles as well as third and fourth ventricles. Ventricular angles are lost (solid arrows) and there is marked dilatation of inferior horns (open arrows).

municating hydrocephalus the radiopharmaceutical should be placed into the lateral ventricles, either directly or by a shunt system that has a two-way valve system in its proximal portion. Subsequent imaging over the distal shunt tip will reveal the presence or absence of shunt obstruction.

In those patients shunted for communicating hydrocephalus, cisternography and distal shunt tip imaging following lumbar puncture has been advocated on the theory that the CSF will follow the pathway of least resistance into the ventricles and out through the shunt. Theoretically, a normal cisternogram in these patients would indicate shunt malfunction. In practice, particularly in infants, Foltz has shown that the aqueduct of Sylvius may occlude after shunting, converting a communicating hydrocephalus into a noncommunicating state (21).

To expedite assessment of a questionably functioning shunt, we often inject the radionuclide directly into the lateral ventricles in both forms of hydrocephalus (Fig. 2-13A). This is preferably done with a 25-gage needle through the self-sealing rubber (silastic) reservoir on the side of the patient's cranium. In patients with one-way valve shunts, the lateral ventricles and proximal portion of the shunt will not be imaged. In these patients the isotope will have to be injected directly into the ventricles for complete shunt evaluation. It is often valuable, however, to inject 1 mCi of pertechnetate into the shunt reservoir (Fig. 2-13B) since in the majority of cases, especially those with dilated ventricles, it is the distal portion of the shunt that is obstructed (Fig. 2-13C, D). After treatment and return to normal or near normal ventricular size, proximal shunt obstruction becomes a more important consideration (22).

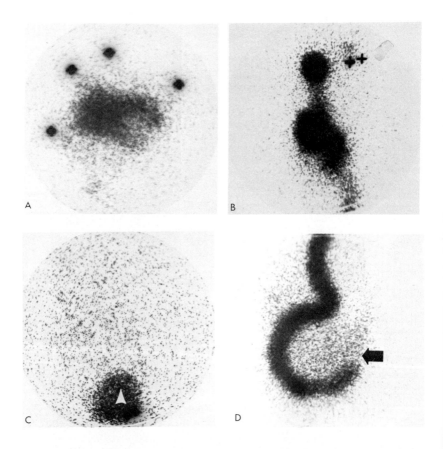

Fig. 2-13. (A) Direct intraventricular injection of radiopharmaceutical in patient with CSF diversionary shunt (markers on calvarium). (B) Because of failure of visualization of radioactivity in distal portion of shunt, there was injection into reservoir of shunt apparatus. This is right lateral view of cranium and upper neck. Radioactivity is seen to be within reservoir of shunt. (C) Abdominal view following injection of radioactivity into shunt reservoir. There is no evidence of radioactivity over distal shunt tip although some radioactivity is seen within urinary bladder (white arrow). This was felt to represent obstruction of shunt, but we were not confident of diagnosis because shunt apparatus itself was not visualized. (D) View of distal shunt after manual pressure causing compression of shunt reservoir. There is expression of radioactivity down into distal shunt tip which allows us to visualize it (arrow), but no definite radioactivity is seen distal to tip of shunt. This was felt to represent obstructed shunt which was later surgically revised.

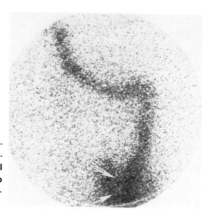

Fig. 2-14. Abdominal image in patient with ventriculoperitoneal shunt with injection into shunt apparatus. Shunt is well visualized as is radioactivity in pool distal to shunt (arrows). This shunt was well-functioning ventriculoperitoneal CSF diversion.

In ventriculovascular shunts, imaging of the distal shunt tip after a lumbar puncture injection is difficult because of the rapid disappearance of the radiopharmaceutical from the distal shunt tip as it enters the circulation. Thus to demonstrate patency of a ventriculoatrial shunt, direct injection of radiopharmaceutical into the lateral cerebral ventricle or the shunt apparatus itself is mandatory. The gamma camera persistence oscilloscope has been very helpful in assessing the patency of these shunts. Additionally, if ^{99m}Tc-pertechnetate is injected into the ventricles and the ventriculovascular shunt is patent, scans of the parotid glands will show activity in 5–30 min. The parotid glands are not visualized for several hours in the presence of an obstructed ventriculovascular shunt (20).

With ventriculoperitoneal shunts, scanning of the distal shunt tip will show a pool of radioactivity in the presence of a functioning shunt (Fig. 2-14). This is very consistent when the radiopharmaceutical is placed in the cerebral ventricle. A definite localized collection of radioactivity has not been observed as consistently when the radionuclide is injected into the lumbar intrathecal space, particularly with radiochelates which are rapidly absorbed in the peritoneal cavity. This is probably because only 50% or less of the radioactivity injected in the spine ever reaches the cranium. Therefore we would not inject a radiopharmaceutical into the lumbar intrathecal space in evaluating possible shunt obstruction unless the status of the subarachnoid CSF pathways is of primary importance. In these instances it is best to determine shunt patency with ^{99m}Tc-pertechnetate initially, followed by conventional cisternography the following day.

Evaluation of CSF Fistula

Openings in the skull associated with discontinuities in the dura provide potential pathways for intracranial infection. These children will often present with recurrent episodes of meningitis. It becomes important in this circumstance to establish the presence and location of a pathway for entry of bacteria into the subarachnoid space. Of the possible methods, radionuclide studies have been the most sensitive and accurate in our experience.

These patients are best imaged with a scintillation camera after injection of radiopharmaceutical into the subarachnoid space. DiChiro and Ashburn (6) have advocated having the patient remain supine until the actual time of imaging to pool the radiopharmaceutical in the basal regions. It is also useful to orient the children in positions that they recognize cause CSF leakage. This history is often obtained from parents when specifically requested.

The most sensitive method of detecting CSF rhinorrhea in our experience is measuring the amount of radioactivity absorbed on appropriately placed cotton pledgets. Quantification by this method is also possible. We use the following technique: Two hours after lumbar intrathecal injection of ^{111}In-DTPA two small neuropatties (0.5-cc-volume special cotton pledgets) are placed in each nostril, one far posteriorly and one superiorly, adjacent to the cribiform plate. These cotton packs are removed after 4 hr and counted for 10 min in a well counter with a window setting of 150–250 keV. The nasal counts are compared with counts obtained from neuropatties placed in the buccal space. Mouth packs are used to provide a background count to allow for any absorption and redistribution of radionuclide from the CSF (23).

We have occasionally encountered patients with small CSF leaks that we could demonstrate by neuropattie counts but could not visualize because the radioactivity outside of the CSF space was not sufficient to form a detectable image.

Quantitative Cisternography

Occasionally patients continue to deteriorate neurologically despite the presence of a functioning CSF shunt. In this circumstance it is appropriate to establish some type of quantitative criterion for the adequacy of shunt function (19, 24). It appears that simply considering the problem of shunt patency as a "yes" or "no" solution is inadequate. Another case in point is the patient who has communicating hydrocephalus without ventricular stasis (those with clearing of ventricles between 24 and 48 hr). These patients apparently are at least partially compensated but as mentioned previously can occasionally decompensate. A method of quantitating CSF flow offers a means of serially monitoring these patients for possible progressive hydrocephalus. Cisternography can be considered essentially as a slow dynamic function study. Assessing the rate of CSF clearance quantitatively (rather than qualitatively as is done at present)

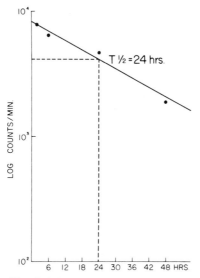

Fig. 2-15. Normal quantitative half-time of radioactivity within subarachnoid space.

offers a method of making finer distinctions between abnormal patterns of CSF flow in patients with both shunted and nonshunted hydrocephalic states.

Akerman (*19*) has described a method to calculate flow of CSF through a shunt by considering both the ventricular volume (measured from rectilinear scans) and the half-time of the injected radiopharmaceutical in the ventricles by the formula: Flow = Volume $\times$ $0.693/T_{1/2}$. Another method using an image display analysis and a computer to generate CSF clearances from regions of interest (e.g., ventricles) has been advocated by DeBlanc (*24*). Harbert and colleagues have generated time-activity curves for total intracranial activity plotted at each scanning interval and expressed as a percent of peak activity. We have used another approach, that of obtaining a $T_{1/2}$ value for the clearance of intracranial activity. The patient is imaged in the routine way at conventional time intervals; 20,000–30,000 counts are obtained, and the average time for four cranial views is computed. Counts per minute versus imaging time intervals are plotted on semilogarithmic paper. After peak activity is reached the data will usually fit a single declining exponential curve from which a $T_{1/2}$ can be obtained after correction for physical decay of the radionuclide. Figure 2-15 shows a time-activity curve for a normal 10 year old. The $T_{1/2}$ is 24 hr.

When shunt malfunction occurs the $T_{1/2}$ invariably increases (Fig. 2-16). This is helpful since we have occasionally observed shunted pa-

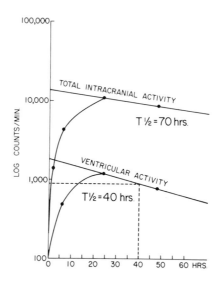

Fig. 2-16. Time-activity curve in patient with partial obstruction of CSF diversionary shunt.

tients whose scans subjectively appeared to resemble their pre-operative scans but their $T_{1/2}$ had changed. Ventricular stasis persisted, and a diagnosis of shunt malfunction was considered. Similar patients have been reported by McCullough and associates (22). When the quantitative curves were obtained in these patients, there was an increase in clearance in the postoperative shunted patients that was not appreciated qualitatively. When patients who were thought to have shunt malfunction had intraventricular pressure measurements made, these determinations were not found to be progressively increasing as expected.

We feel that quantitative cisternography and ventriculography may provide an objective method of analysis that has considerable potential in predicting the efficacy of CSF drainage procedures in patients with hydrocephalus. Individual patients can be serially evaluated, and finer distinctions can be made between normal and abnormal CSF dynamics than are presently possible with qualitative techniques.

Thus radionuclide imaging studies will provide clinically useful information in children with abnormalities of CSF movement and absorption. We would again emphasize that not only are the diagnostic considerations different from adults but the technical ones are also. Further use of this diagnostic test in children with neurological problems is anticipated.

Acknowledgments

Many members of the Department of Radiology and Radiological Sciences, especially the Division of Nuclear Medicine contributed to this chapter. The scans were made in the Division of Nuclear Medicine under the direction of Henry N. Wagner, Jr., and the graphs in the Department of Art as Applied to Medicine. The Fellows in Nuclear Medicine assisted in collecting the cases. The research in CSF dynamics was supported by the James Picker Foundation, NAS-NRC.

References

1. JAMES AE, MATHEWS ES, DeBLANC HG, et al: Cerebrospinal fluid imaging: its current status. *J Can Assoc Radiol* 23: 157–167, 1972

2. HARBERT JC: Radionuclide cisternography. *Semin Nucl Med* 1: 90–106, 1971

3. McCULLOUGH DC, HARBERT JC: Pediatric radionuclide cisternography. *Semin Nucl Med* 2: 343–352, 1972

4. McCULLOUGH DC, HARBERT JC, MIALE A, et al: Radioisotope cisternography in the evaluation of hydrocephalus in infancy and childhood. *Radiology* 102: 645–652, 1972

5. JAMES AE, NEW PF, HEINZ ER, et al: A cisternographic classification of hydrocephalus. *Am J Roentgenol Radium Ther Nucl Med* 115: 39–44, 1972

6. DiCHIRO G, ASHBURN WL: Radioisotope cisternography, ventriculography and myelographs. In *Nuclear Medicine,* 2nd ed, Blahd WH, ed, New York, McGraw-Hill, 1972

7. DiCHIRO G: Movement of the cerebrospinal fluid in human beings. *Nature* 204: 290–291, 1964

8. JAMES AE, HURLEY PJ, HELLER RM, et al: CSF imaging (cisternography) in pediatric patient. *Ann Radiol* 14: 591–600, 1971

9. ALKER GJ, GLASAUER FE, LESLIE EV: Isotope cisternography and ventriculography in hydrocephalus of children. In *Cisternography and Hydrocephalus.* Harbert JC, ed, Springfield, Ill, C C Thomas, 1972, pp 385–396

10. CONWAY JJ: Dynamic studies in pediatric nuclear medicine. In *Clinical Dynamic Function Studies with Radionuclides.* Croll MC, ed, New York, Appleton-Century-Crofts, 1972, pp 233–252

11. KEREIAKES JG, WELLMAN HN, TIEMAN J, et al: Radiopharmaceutical dosimetry in pediatrics. *Radiology* 90: 925–930, 1968

12. CONWAY JJ: Consideration for the performance of radionuclide procedures in children. *Semin Nucl Med* 2: 311–315, 1972

13. HOSAIN F, SOM P, JAMES AE, et al: Radioactive chelates for cisternography: the basis and the choice. In *Cisternography and Hydrocephalus.* Harbert JC, ed, Springfield, Ill, C C Thomas, 1972, pp 185–193

14. GILDAY DL: Personal communication, 1973

15. LARSON SM, SCHALL GL, DiCHIRO G: The unsuccessful injection in cisternography: incidence, cause, and appearance. In *Cisternography and Hydrocephalus.* Harbert JC, ed, Springfield, Ill, C C Thomas, 1972, pp 153–160

16. KIRSCHNER PJ: Personal communication, 1972

17. HAKIM S, ADAMS RD: The special clinical problem of symptomatic hydrocephalus with normal cerebrospinal fluid pressure. *J Neurol Neurosurg and Psych* 2: 307–327, 1965

18. McCullough DC, Harbert JC, Luessenhop AJ: Pediatric hydrocephalus: Contributions of radioisotope cisternography to diagnosis and management. In *Cisternography and Hydrocephalus.* Harbert JC, ed, Springfield, Ill, C C Thomas, 1972, pp 375–383

19. Akerman M, de Tovar G, Guist G: Radioisotope ventriculography and cisternography in non-communicating hydrocephalus. In *Cisternography and Hydrocephalus.* Harbert JC, ed, Springfield, Ill, C C Thomas, 1972, pp 483–501

20. DiChiro G, Grove AS: Evaluation of surgical and spontaneous CSF shunts by isotope scanning. *J Neurosurg* 24: 743–748, 1966

21. Foltz EL, Shurtleff DB: Conversion of communicating hydrocephalus to non-communicating hydrocephalus secondary to stenosis or occlusion of the aqueduct during ventricular shunts. *J Neurosurg* 24: 520–529, 1966

22. McCullough DC, Fox JL, Curl FD, et al: Effects of CSF shunts on intracranial pressure and CSF dynamics. In *Cisternography and Hydrocephalus.* Harbert JC, ed, Springfield, Ill, C C Thomas, 1972, pp 355–342

23. McKusick K: Personal communication, 1974

24. DeBlanc HJ, Natarajan TK, James AE, et al: Computer assisted quantitative cisternography and ventriculography. In *Cisternography and Hydrocephalus.* Harbert JC, ed, Springfield, Ill, C C Thomas, 1972, pp 471–482

Discussion

Daniel Schere (Children's Hospital, Buenos Aires, Argentina): In ventricular entry and normal size ventricles how are you sure of which image corresponds to the lateral ventricle?

Dr. James: In our experience of over 500 cisternograms, with a lumbar injection, radiopharmaceutical does not enter normal-sized ventricles to the extent that they can be imaged. We believe that this is due to the net current of flow from the choroid plexus of the ventricles to the arachnoid villi in the parasagittal region (*1*). When ventricles become enlarged and the ependymal lining allows greater migration of CSF constituents, the ventricular entry of the radiopharmaceutical is seen. We believe this process may be responsible for the current of flow outward from the ventricles (James AE, Strecker EP, Sperber E, et al: An alternative pathway of cerebrospinal fluid absorption in communicating hydrocephalus transependymal movement. *Radiology* 111(1): 143–146, 1974).

Dr. Schere: Is there any way of determining patency of a ventriculoatrial shunt by lumbar tap?

Dr. James: I would assume that you mean instilling radiopharmaceutical at the time of lumbar puncture. One can then examine the entire shunt system since the radiopharmaceutical will enter the ventricle if a communicating hydrocephalus exists. If there is a noncommunicating hydrocephalus the patency or obstruction of peripheral pathway can be confirmed.

Jay S. Budin (Kaiser Permanente Medical Center, Sacramento,

Calif.): Are cisternographic techniques of value in diagnosis of pseudo-tumor cerebri and predicting whether hydrocephalus will arrest?

Dr. James: There are basically two findings reported with cisternog-raphy in pseudotumor cerebri. The first is a delayed transfer of the radio-pharmaceutical from the subarachnoid space and the other is a persist-ence of the radioactivity in the parasagittal region. We collected the cisternograms from our institution, the University of Florida, the Univer-sity of Chicago, and Georgetown University to examine the patterns and found them to be normal. The delay in transfer was confirmed (James AE, Harbert JC, Hoffer PB, et al: CSF imaging in pseudotumor cerebri. *J Neurol Neurosurg Psychiatry,* in press). At present CSF imaging does not appear to be clinically useful in evaluating patients with pseudotumor cerebri but may offer some insight as to the pathophysiology and will exclude alternative diagnoses.

To answer the second part of your question, Alker, Glasauer, and Leslie studied 25 patients with arrested hydrocephalus. They found ven-tricular entry with stasis but decided not to shunt the patients on clinical grounds. This has been our experience also. Why there is no progression of hydrocephalus or the neurological signs are stable is unknown. We have observed transependymal migration of radiopharmaceutical in com-municating hydrocephalus in dogs and nonhuman primates (Strecker EP, James AE: The evaluation of CSF flow and absorption: clinical and ex-perimental studies. *Neuroradiol* 6: 200–205, 1973. James AE, Strecker EP, Novak GR, et al: Correlation of serial cisternograms and CSF pres-sure measurements in experimental communicating hydrocephalus. *Neurology* 23: 1226–1233, 1973. Strecker EP, James AE, Konigsmark B, et al: Autoradiographic observations in experimental hydrocephalus. *Acta Neurol* 24: 192–197, 1974. Strecker EP, Kelly JET, Scheffel U, et al: CSF absorption in communicating hydrocephalus: Evaluation of radioactive albumin from subarachnoid space to plasma. *Neurology* 23: 854–864, 1973). This may form an alternative pathway of CSF absorp-tion and "compensate" for the original abnormality.

Chapter **3**

Thyroid

Delbert A. Fisher and Delores E. Johnson

The spectrum of thyroid disease in childhood and adolescence has been altered significantly during the past two decades. Before 1960 thyroid dysgenesis, inborn abnormalities in thyroid hormone synthesis and metabolism, juvenile thyrotoxicosis, and physiological goiter of adolescence accounted for most of the diagnosed thyroid disorders in the pediatric age group. In the interim we have become aware that the majority of patients with adolescent goiters either have chronic lymphocytic (Hashimoto's) thyroiditis or nontoxic diffuse goiters, often referred to as simple colloid goiters. Recent data suggest that as many as 1.3% of school children in the United States may suffer from Hashimoto's thyroiditis (*1*), and relative-incidence data suggest that simple colloid goiter may occur in 1% of adolescents (*2, 3*). Thus, in order of frequency, thyroid disorders in childhood and adolescence include Hashimoto's thyroiditis, simple colloid goiter, juvenile thyrotoxicosis, congenital thyroid dysgenesis, and inborn defects in thyroid hormone synthesis or metabolism. Less common disorders include acute (subacute) nonsuppurative thyroiditis (which is probably a viral thyroiditis), suppurative thyroiditis, functional and nonfunctional thyroid nodules, and thyroid carcinoma. The most important approaches to diagnosis of thyroid disorders in childhood and adolescence include the history and physical examination supplemented by selected in vitro function tests (See Chapter 14). These approaches recently have been reviewed (*4, 5*). In certain instances in vivo thyroid function testing can be useful in the differential diagnosis of thyroid disease in childhood, and it is this area with which the present discussion will deal.

Thyroid Physiology

Basic aspects of thyroid follicular cell function are illustrated in Fig. 3-1. Inorganic iodide in blood is "trapped" or actively transported into the cell against a concentration gradient of 10–30 to 1. This iodide is transported to the follicular cell surface and oxidized, probably to iodine, under the influence of a thyroid peroxidase. The iodine then reacts with tyrosine residues already incorporated in molecules of newly synthesized thyroglobulin. The tyrosine is sequentially iodinated to monoiodotyrosine (MIT) and diiodotyrosine (DIT). Molecules of MIT and DIT appropriately situated sterically in the thyroglobulin molecule are coupled, probably enzymatically, as follows:

$$DIT + DIT - alanine = tetraiodothyronine \text{ (thyroxine or } T_4)$$

$$MIT + DIT - alanine = triiodothyronine \text{ } (T_3).$$

Many of the MIT and DIT molecules remain uncoupled, however, so that follicular colloid is composed of thyroglobulin containing large amounts of uncoupled MIT and DIT as well as T_3 and T_4. Under the stimulus of TSH (Fig. 3-2) the stored thyroglobulin is reincorporated into the follicular cell as colloid droplets by a process of endocytosis. Each engulfed colloid "droplet" merges with a lysosome to form a phagolysosome, and the thyroglobulin molecule is broken down by proteolytic enzymes as this droplet-lysosome packet is transported to the plasma membrane surface of the cell. Here the MIT, DIT, T_4, and T_3 are released. The T_4 and T_3 diffuse rapidly into the blood stream; the MIT and DIT are deiodinated under the influence of an iodotyrosine deiodinase and the iodide recycled again through the organification process.

Choice of Nuclides

In vivo thyroid function testing is conducted with isotopes of iodine, the rate-limiting substrate for thyroidal hormonogenesis, or with pertechnetate, an anion which the thyroid follicular cells will concentrate or "trap" similarly to iodide, but will not organify. Table 3-1 summarizes the physical characteristics of these isotopes, their advantages or indications, their disadvantages, and the average radiation dose to the thyroid in the infant, child, and adult. The latter is expressed as estimated dose in rads per microcurie administered assuming an uptake of 27% and a biological half-life of 68 days. For many years the "standard" isotope for thyroid studies has been [131]I. This isotope, however, has the disadvantage of a high radiation dose to the gland, especially in infants and children. Furthermore the high-energy gamma ray (364 keV) requires low-efficiency, thick septal collimators for scanning. More recently ^{125}I, ^{123}I, and ^{99m}Tc-pertechnetate have been used to reduce radiation to the patient. The low-energy gamma rays (35 keV) of ^{125}I prevent its use for routine uptake studies. However, it has an advantage for scanning because it is used with thin septal collimators which give three times more counts per micro-curie of tracer and thus produce good scans in children. Because pertechnetate is not organified, it can be used only for early uptake or "trapping" studies (3–20 min) and for early scanning. The isotope of choice in

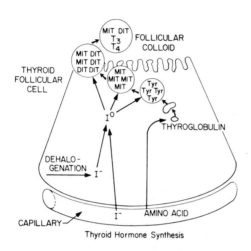

Thyroid Hormone Synthesis

Fig. 3-1. Steps in thyroid hormone synthesis and storage. See text for details.

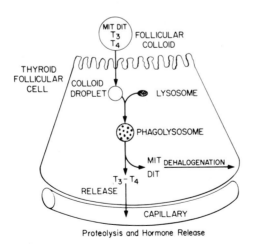

Proteolysis and Hormone Release

Fig. 3-2. Steps in thyroid hormone release. See text for details.

TABLE 3-1. Radioactive Tracers for In Vivo Thyroid Diagnosis

	^{131}I	^{125}I	$^{99m}TcO_4^-$	^{123}I	^{132}I
Emission	Beta, gamma	Gamma (E.C.)	Gamma	Gamma (E.C.)	Beta, gamma
Source	Reactor, fission	Reactor	Generator	Accelerator	Generator
Energy (keV)	364	35	140	159	670, 760
Tissue half-thickness (cm)	6.3	1.8	4.7	4.7	8.1, 8.6
Half-life	8.1 days	60.6 days	6 hr	13.3 hr	2.3 hr
Radiation dose* Infant	5.0	0.5	<0.001	0.06	0.05
Child	2.5	0.8	<0.001	0.04	0.03
Adult	1.5	1.0	<0.001	0.02	0.01
Collimator	Thick septal	Thin septal	Thin septal and camera	Thin septal and camera	—
Indications	1. Routine and special uptake studies 2. Following TSH stimulation or T_3 suppression to compare with routine ^{125}I scan 3. Whole-body scanning following ^{131}I Rx for thyroid Ca	1. Routine scanning	1. 20-min uptake 2. Scanning of infants and children	1. Routine uptake and scanning	1. 20-min uptakes 2. Serial uptakes following TSH stimulation or T_3 suppression
Disadvantages	1. Low efficiency 2. High radiation dose	1. Low energy	1. Trapping only 2. High background	1. Higher cost 2. Cyclotron produced	1. Very short half-life 2. Many high-energy gammas

* Rads to thyroid per microcurie given assuming RAI uptake of 27% and biological half-life of 68 days.

children is ^{123}I. It has all of the advantages of ^{131}I and, in addition, minimizes the dose of radiation to the thyroid. Its gamma-ray energy is nearly ideal for imaging. This isotope is cyclotron-produced and relatively expensive, but increasing use should lower the cost.

Thyroid Uptake

Thyroid uptake studies can be conducted very early, early, or late. Very early (3–20 min) uptake studies measure the activity of the thyroid follicular cell iodide-trapping mechanism and usually are not routine. Early uptake studies (2–6 hr) measure predominantly iodide trapping and organification. Late uptake studies measure predominantly organification and release of organic iodine. The rate of thyroidal iodine uptake is inversely related to iodine intake which has increased markedly in the United States during the past two decades (6). Thus the mean thyroidal radioiodine uptake has decreased in most areas so that uptake tests are not useful in distinguishing euthyroid and hypothyroid subjects. Moreover, mean thyroidal radioiodine uptake is quite variable geographically so that normal values must be locally established (6). In general the mean 24-hr uptake varies from 15 to 30%. (See Appendix, Table A-7 for uptake data in children. Uptake in the newborn and very young children is much higher.) The 2-hr uptake usually approximates 25% and the 6-hr uptake 50% of the 24-hr value.

There are many variations in uptake methodology, but in general uptake is measured with a directional scintillation counter. Corrections usually are made for background activity by recounting with a lead shield over the patient's neck; the difference between the shielded and unshielded counts represents the radioactivity in the gland. This is then expressed as a percentage of the dose given by counting the dose in a neck phantom. Neck background also can be corrected by subtracting knee activity from gross neck counts. For infants and small children a lead adapter is inserted into the collimator to reduce the field of view and exclude the upper thorax and head. The test dose usually is given orally to a fasting patient. The lag time for an oral dose compared with an intravenous dose in nonfasting adult subjects is 15–20 min (7). Thus the radioiodine dose for very early uptake studies is given intravenously.

An overactive gland accumulates more radioactive iodine than normal, and an underactive gland less. There is a good deal of overlap between uptake in euthyroid and hypothyroid subjects so that in vitro tests discriminate these groups more accurately than uptake tests. Uptake studies are most useful in the diagnosis of thyrotoxicosis and inborn or acquired defects in thyroid hormone synthesis or metabolism. In thyrotoxicosis radioiodine is trapped rapidly, and both the rates of organification and release are increased. In addition, the rate of uptake usually is

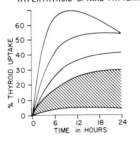

Fig. 3-3. Representative patterns of thyroidal radioiodine uptake. Shaded area represents usual range of early and late uptake throughout most of United States. However, normal values must be locally determined. In hypothyroid subjects both early and late uptake may be reduced or normal. In hyperactive glands, represented by upper three lines, both early and late uptake may be increased. With marked, prolonged thyroid gland stimulation associated with rapid release, early uptake may exceed late uptake value as in upper line.

increased to a greater extent than the percentage uptake so that early uptake tests are most discriminating. Rapid release may further reduce the 24-hr uptake relative to the 2–6-hr uptakes (Fig. 3-3). Thus measurements of both early and late uptake are desirable.

In patients with inborn or acquired defects in thyroid hormone synthesis, both the early and late uptake values also are increased. With prolonged, marked overstimulation of the gland associated with thyroid iodine depletion, early uptake tends to be increased relatively more than the late uptake values, and the difference between early and late results decreases. This pattern of increased early uptake and relatively or absolutely lower late uptake (Fig. 3-3) may occur because of an increased rate of thyroidal organic iodine release and/or defective organification of iodine with early release of nonorganified iodide. To differentiate these possibilities the perchlorate discharge test has been devised.

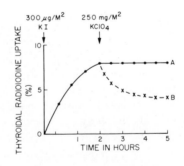

Fig. 3-4. Perchlorate discharge test. See text for details.

In normal subjects perchlorate ion competes with iodide for trapping by the thyroid follicular cell plasma membrane. Thus the administration of 10 mg/kg or 250 mg/m² oral potassium perchlorate 60–120 min after administration of a tracer dose of radioiodine rapidly inhibits or blocks iodide trapping with the result that thyroidal radioiodine uptake (content) plateaus within 5–10 min (Fig. 3-4). Some of the perchlorate is transported intracellularly and competes with iodide for intracellular binding sites. Normally intracellular iodide is rapidly oxidized and organified so that it is not "displaced" by perchlorate. However, if there is a defect in the organification system, the intracellular perchlorate displaces nonorganified (inorganic) iodide and a perchlorate discharge occurs. When this discharge is in excess of 10% of the total gland radioiodine measured at the time of perchlorate administration, the discharge is considered abnormal.

Takeuchi and associates have shown that the sensitivity and usefulness of the test are enhanced by administering 15 μg/kg or 300 μg/m² of potassium iodide at the time of radioiodine administration (8). This iodide-perchlorate discharge test and the perchlorate discharge test are particularly useful as diagnostic aids in patients with goitrous hypothyroidism due to a defective peroxidase system and those with Hashimoto's thyroiditis. However, positive tests also can occur in patients with iodide-induced goiter, in patients following administration of goitrogens, and in thyrotoxic patients, especially following radioiodine therapy. A typical positive discharge test in a patient with goitrous hypothyroidism due to an inborn defect in organification of iodine is shown in Fig. 3-5. A positive discharge test in an adolescent female with Hashimoto's thyroiditis is shown in Fig. 3-6.

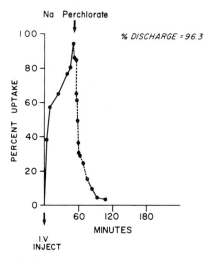

Fig. 3-5. Positive perchlorate discharge test in child with inborn thyroidal organification defect.

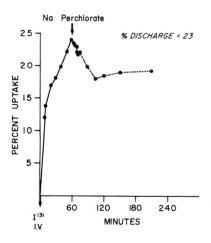

Fig. 3-6. Positive perchlorate discharge test in adolescent girl with Hashimoto's thyroiditis.

Thyroid Scans

Thyroid scans are useful for localizing ectopic thyroid tissue and for structure-function correlation studies of the thyroid gland. The latter include localization of hyperfunctioning and nonfunctioning thyroid nodules and delineation of the irregular patterns of distribution of thyroidal radioiodine which occur in thyroid dysgenesis and in Hashimoto's (chronic lymphocytic) thyroiditis. Scintillation cameras and minicomputers amplify the usefulness of such examinations with short-lived isotopes and reduce the radiation dose to the patient (9). Figure 3-7 shows a typical neck scan in a patient with thyroid dysgenesis and ectopic thyroid tissue near the base of the tongue. Figures 3-8–3-12 show the types of abnormal scans observed in patients with Hashimoto's thyroiditis. Since this disease is

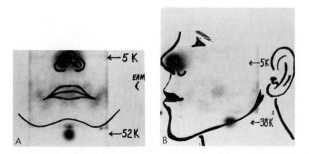

Fig. 3-7. Frontal (A) and lateral views (B) of typical neck scan in patient with thyroid dysgenesis and residual ectopic thyroid tissue near base of tongue. Numbers refer to relative intensities of radiation. Midline inframandibular radioiodine activity represents thyroid tissue.

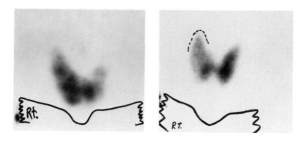

Fig. 3-8. (Left) Typical thyroid scan in patient with Hashimoto's thyroiditis showing "hill and valley" pattern of irregular areas of increased density separated by areas of relatively lesser density.

Fig. 3-9. (Right) Common scan pattern in patient with Hashimoto's thyroiditis in which entire lobe or part of lobe shows pattern of relatively diminished density. Other lobe also is usually abnormal.

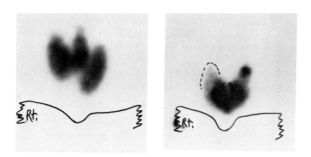

Fig. 3-10. (Left) Thyroid scan in patient with Hashimoto's thyroiditis and enlarged, thickened, and ropy pyramidal lobe. Abnormal pyramidal lobe also shows "hill and valley" pattern of radioiodine distribution.

Fig. 3-11. (Right) Thyroid scan showing prominent, nodular isthmus with irregular radioiodine distribution in patient with Hashimoto's thyroiditis.

usually progressive, the scan pattern may be quite variable. Early in the disease scans may show a fairly uniform density distribution pattern. However, the most common scan pattern depicts irregular foci of increased density separated by lighter areas, giving a "hill and valley" appearance (Fig. 3-8). This is in contrast to the "moth eaten" or "Swiss cheese" appearance of multinodular goiter. Another common scan pattern shows an entire lobe or part of a lobe to have uniformly diminished density whereas this lobe on palpation feels firmer than the other lobe and has discrete borders which do not blend with adjacent neck tissue (Fig. 3-9). By contrast, simple diffuse goiters show increased density over the thickest areas of the gland. An enlarged, thickened, ropy pyramidal lobe (Fig. 3-10) and a prominent isthmus (Fig. 3-11) are often visualized in

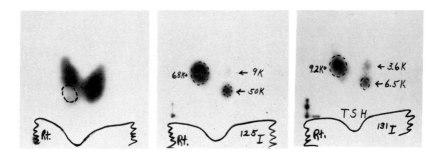

Fig. 3-12. (Left) Relatively cold nodule in patient with Hashimoto's thyroiditis.

Fig. 3-13. (Middle) Initial thyroid scan in adolescent with bilateral functioning thyroid nodules. Numbers indicate relative radiation intensities. 9K area is minimal activity detectable in normal left lobe tissue.

Fig. 3-14. (Right) Thyroid scan in patient in Fig. 3-13 after exogenous TSH administration. Again numbers indicate relative radiation intensities. Suppressed left lobe tissue now is visible.

scans of patients with Hashimoto's disease. Finally the disease may present as a hypofunctioning "cold" nodule (Fig. 3-12).

Figures 3-13 and 3-14 show the usefulness of thyroid scanning in an adolescent with two hyperfunctioning thyroid nodules. The patient was mildly thyrotoxic and presented with two discrete nodules, each approximately 1 × 2 cm in size. The initial scan showed uptake in the nodules and little or no uptake in the surrounding thyroid tissue. After stimulation by an exogenous dose of 10 units TSH, uptake in the normal thyroid tissue surrounding the nodules was observed, indicating that the nodules were functioning autonomously and suppressing normal thyroid function.

Other Tests

Several special test procedures find occasional usefulness. The T_3 suppression test has been used as a confirmatory test for the diagnosis of thyrotoxicosis when the in vitro function tests show borderline results (*10*). The test is conducted by measuring radioiodine uptake, administering 1.5 μg T_3/kg/24 hr for 7 days and repeating the uptake measurement. It is essential that the T_3 be given for 7 days. Failure of suppression of thyroid uptake to 50% or less of the initial value indicates autonomy of thyroidal function, a characteristic of thyrotoxicosis. Recent improvements in quality and quantity of in vitro function tests, particularly the radioimmunoassay of serum T_3, have reduced the number of patients in the borderline area so that suppression testing now is less frequently necessary. Moreover, the 7-day course of exogenous T_3 in a thyrotoxic patient may produce undesirable side effects. Finally the thyroid-releasing hormone (TRH) response test, measuring serum TSH in response to TRH, is a more convenient test and may turn out to be reliable for the confirmation of thyrotoxicosis (*11, 12*).

The TSH stimulation test has long been used as a test of thyroid function, particularly to assess thyroid reserve and to differentiate primary and secondary hypothyroidism (*9*). The test is rarely indicated in present day thyroid diagnosis. The TRH stimulation test more reliably differentiates primary and secondary hypothyroidism, and the serum TSH measurement and TRH stimulation tests are better indicators of thyroid functional reserve (*13–15*).

References

1. RALLISON ML, DOBYNS BM, KEATING FR, et al: Diagnosis and maternal history of thyroiditis in children. *Pediatr Res* 6: 355, 1972

2. LING SM, KAPLAN SA, WEITZMAN JJ, et al: Euthyroid goiters in children: correlation of needle biopsy with other clinical and laboratory findings in chronic lymphocytic thyroiditis and simple goiter. *Pediatrics* 44: 695–708, 1969

3. GREENBERG AH, CZERNICHOW P, HUNG W, et al: Juvenile lymphocytic thyroiditis: clinical laboratory and histological correlations. *J Clin Endocrinol Metab* 30: 293–301, 1970

4. FISHER DA: Advances in laboratory diagnosis of thyroid disease, Part I. *J Pediatr* 82: 1–9, 1973

5. FISHER DA: Advances in laboratory diagnosis of thyroid disease, Part II. *J Pediatr* 82: 187–191, 1973

6. ODDIE TH, FISHER DA, MCCONAHEY WM, et al: Iodine intake in the United States: A reassessment. *J Clin Endocrinol Metab* 30: 659–665, 1971

7. ODDIE TH, FISHER DA, CRINER G: Lag time for oral radioiodide tracer doses. *J Clin Endocrinol Metab* 26: 581–582, 1966

8. TAKEUCHI K, SUZUKI H, HORIUCHI Y, et al: Significance of iodide-perchlorate discharge test for detection of iodine organification defect of the thyroid. *J Clin Endocrinol Metab* 31: 144–146, 1970

9. HURLEY PJ, MAISEY MN, NATARAJAN TK, et al: A computerized system for rapid evaluation of thyroid function. *J Clin Endocrinol Metab* 34: 354–360, 1972

10. HARDEN RM: Quantitative isotopic tests of thyroid function including tests of thyroid homeostasis, In *The Thyroid,* 3rd ed, Werner SC, Ingbar SH, eds, New York, Harper and Row, 1971, pp 193–214

11. LAWTON NF, EKINS RP, NABARRO JDN: Failure of pituitary response to thyrotropin-releasing hormones in euthyroid Graves' disease. *Lancet* 2: 14–16, 1971

12. ORMSTON BJ, GARRY R, CRYER RJ, et al: Thyrotropin-releasing hormone as a test of thyroid function. *Lancet* 2: 10–14, 1971

13. ANDERSON MS, BOWERS CY, KASTIN AJ, et al: Synthetic thyrotropin releasing hormone. A potent stimulator of thyrotropin secretion in man. *N Engl J Med* 285: 1279–1283, 1971

14. FOLEY TR, OWINGS J, HAYFORD JT, et al: Serum thyrotropin-releasing hormone in normal children and hypopituitary patients. *J Clin Invest* 51: 431–437, 1972

15. Costom BH, Grumbach MM, Kaplan SL: Effect of thyrotropin releasing factor on serum thyroid-stimulating hormone. *J Clin Invest* 50: 2219–2225, 1971

Discussion

Brian M. Buchea (University of New Mexico, Albuquerque, N.M.): Is there anything new on ^{131}I therapy of 10–11 year olds with Graves' disease?

Dr. Fisher: There still is controversy about treating children or adolescents with thyrotoxicosis with radioiodine. We do not like to treat patients under 20 years of age with radioiodine but consider this on rare occasion between 14 or 15 and 20 years. And we avoid surgery. Thus usually we treat with antithyroid drugs. We treat 3–6 months beyond the time the thyroid gland returns to normal size (and the patient is euthyroid), after which time we try the patient off medication.

Julian R. Karelitz (Saint John's Hospital, Santa Monica, Calif.): You classified a euthyroid patient with a nonsuppressible autonomously functioning multinodular goiter as having Plummer's disease. By definition, should not a patient with Plummer's disease be toxic? Was this patient a T_3 secreter?

Dr. Fisher: Dr. Plummer initially described toxic patients with nodule(s). But most hyperfunctioning nodules probably do not secrete enough hormone to produce toxicity. The nodule has to secrete more hormone than the thyroid gland normally does to produce clinical thyrotoxicosis. Lesser amounts will merely suppress the normally functioning gland. Thus at least some thyroidologists now refer to both functioning nodules which suppress the normal gland as well as those which produce clinical toxicity as Plummer's disease. This patient's serum T_3 concentration was normal.

Chapter **4**

Lung

Gerald L. DeNardo, Willard J. Blankenship, John A. Burdine, Jr., and Sally J. DeNardo

Conventional pulmonary function studies are a valuable tool in the management of the adult patient with lung disease. Because of difficulty of performance and lack of reliable standards for the rapidly maturing pediatric patient, however, pulmonary evaluation has been limited primarily to the chest x-ray, blood gas measurements, and in some cases, measurement of carbon monoxide diffusion capacity. Other more sophisticated and tedious tests are available only in a research setting. To improve the diagnosis and treatment of lung disorders in neonates, infants, and children, better methods for evaluation of pulmonary function are needed. Much information can be obtained from radionuclide ventilation and perfusion studies, which can be performed in any age group including the premature infant. A brief review of lung development and growth is necessary to better understand the role of these techniques.

Fetal and Postnatal Development

In the 24-day embryo the lung begins as an outpouching of the gut. Two primary branches of the primitive lung bud, destined to become the major bronchi, appear at 28 days and by 12 weeks segmental branching has reached about 25 divisions so that the lobes of the lung are well defined. From the 16th to the 25th week canalization of the glandular elements occurs and mucous glands and cartilagenous structures proliferate. Capillaries arise from the mesenchymal tissue.

From 24 to 28 weeks and into postnatal life, alveoli appear from alveolar ducts, respiratory passages elongate, and capillaries proliferate around terminal air spaces. Although the alveolar septa are still thickened, it becomes possible for the first time for the alveolar-capillary membrane to sufficiently exchange gases to support life. Surfactant production by alveolar cells improves the stability of the lung.

The fetal lung contains much secreted fluid and is collapsed in utero. Before birth the pulmonary vascular resistance is greater than that in the systemic circulation, and much of the blood flow is diverted away from the lung through the patent ductus arteriosus and foramen ovale. The expansion of the lungs during the first breath produces a decrease in pulmonary vascular resistance and a tenfold increase of pulmonary blood flow. There is closure of the foramen ovale and the ductus arteriosus by 18 hr of age in the full term, healthy neonate.

The anatomic growth of the lung proceeds in a uniform manner whether the fetus is in utero or delivered prematurely. During the first 5–8 years of life, the diameter of the trachea triples, alveolar dimensions increase about fourfold, and alveolar numbers increase by a factor of 10. The relatively large airways tend to facilitate the movement of air even though they also result in greater wasted ventilation. Although more subject to collapse, the smaller alveoli offer a greater surface area for gaseous exchange. However, the metabolism of the infant per kilogram of body weight is nearly twice that of an adult so that the infant has less pulmonary reserve than the adult. By 8 years of life the lung resembles its adult counterpart and conventional pulmonary function tests are applicable.

Pulmonary Function by Scintigraphy

The primary and vital function of the lung is the exchange of oxygen for carbon dioxide. This is accomplished by an appropriate distribution of the pulmonary arterial blood flowing through the lungs and the air ventilating the lungs. Insofar as this distribution is matched on a one-to-one basis, efficient gas exchange occurs. Regional uncoupling of ventilation and perfusion is present in many diseases of the lung and results in inefficient exchange of gases. Such nonuniform matching of ventilation and perfusion may occur in a lung, a lobe, a segment, a region of a segment, or even at the alveolar level. Radionuclide techniques are the only routine clinical methods for assessing uniformity of matching since they allow independent measurement of regional ventilation and perfusion; these techniques do not detect nonuniformity at the alveolar level. The pediatric patient benefits uniquely from these procedures because they are reasonably simple and atraumatic and can be accomplished without patient cooperation in contrast to conventional pulmonary function studies (1–3).

A variety of radionuclide studies of pulmonary function are available (Table 4-1) (4, 5). Regional blood flow is monitored with radioactive particles (e.g., ^{99m}Tc-macroaggregated albumin) which are injected in a

TABLE 4-1.   Scintigraphic Studies of the Lung

Ventilation
    Radioactive aerosols?
    Radioactive gases
        Soluble
        Insoluble
Perfusion
    Particulate blockade
    Radioactive gases
        Soluble
        Insoluble

TABLE 4-2.   Use of ^{133}Xe in Lung Studies

Perfusion—static distribution after i.v. xenon
Ventilation
    Ventilated alveoli—static distribution after single breath Xe, after rebreathing Xe;
        dynamic washout rate of inspired Xe
    Perfused alveoli—dynamic washout rate of i.v. Xe
Lung volume—static distribution after rebreathing Xe

peripheral vein with subsequent trapping by the pulmonary capillary bed. The distribution of radioactivity reflects the relative distribution of blood flowing through the lungs (6). Radioactive gases in solution can also be used for this purpose. The most commonly used radionuclide at present is poorly soluble ^{133}Xe which may be used to assess regional perfusion and ventilation to the lungs in several ways (Table 4-2).

Ventilation can be assessed by the inhalation of aerosolized particles, but since the distribution of particles depends on other factors in addition to ventilation, these studies are more appropriately referred to as "inhalation lung studies" (5). Radioactive gases provide a more physiologic measurement of regional ventilation. Regional ventilation can be measured by static imaging of the distribution of ^{133}Xe during breath-holding following single-breath inhalation. For a more dynamic, and possibly more physiologic index, gas clearance may be determined by sequential imaging of the washout of injected or inhaled gas (7).

In adults or children a combination of these studies is usually done, and the lung imaging technique consists of administering:

1. radioactive particles intravenously to determine regional perfusion, and
2. ^{133}Xe gas by inhalation for the measurement of ventilation.

In infants, however, ventilation may be more easily measured by another technique. When ^{133}Xe dissolved in saline is injected into a peripheral vein, the initial distribution in the lungs reflects regional perfusion. Since xenon is insoluble, 95% passes into the alveoli on the first pulmonary circulation. As the infant breathes normal ambient air, the ^{133}Xe is cleared from the alveoli, and the rate of washout becomes a measure of regional ventilation. After an injection or single breath of ^{133}Xe, the region of greatest radioactivity is the best perfused or ventilated lung, but on the washout study a relative *increase* in radioactivity indicates an area of *decreased* ventilation in the lung.

Finally, if the individual rebreathes the radioactive gas from a closed system to the point of an equilibrium concentration, the radioactivity in any given region will reflect the relative functioning lung volume of that area. This is a very important item of information because it provides an in vivo method of calibration which facilitates quantification and separates functioning from nonfunctioning air space. The washout rate of equilibrated gas can be followed as before.

Instrumentation and Radiopharmaceuticals

A stationary imaging device such as the Anger gamma scintillation camera is necessary for ventilation and perfusion scintigraphy in the pediatric patient. A parallel-hole collimator is suitable for studies of older children, but some method of magnifying the very small lungs of infants and neonates is necessary. A converging collimator is ideal, although a pinhole collimator may be used with some reduction of efficiency. Low-energy collimators are appropriately used with ^{99m}Tc-macroaggregates or microspheres, ^{133}Xe, or ^{125}Xe. These radiopharmaceuticals are particularly advantageous because of their high photon flux per unit of radiation dose. In addition, the newer ^{125}Xe provides a more optimum photon energy than ^{133}Xe. Particles labeled with ^{131}I or ^{113m}In require high-energy collimators and have undesirable physical characteristics, particularly in the young child.

Clinical Conditions

Normal pulmonary scintigraphy. Mediastinal structures, such as the heart, appear as regions of reduced radioactivity on both anterior and posterior views (Fig. 4-1). The diaphragm, not well defined on the anterior and posterior views, is often better delineated on lateral views (8).

Hyaline membrane disease. This disorder develops in premature infants because of a lack of production and release of surfactant. Atelectasis, which is present in utero, persists or quickly redevelops after birth, and leads to hypoxemia and a reduction in pulmonary blood flow. There may be a persistence of both the ductus arteriosus and the foramen ovale with right-to-left shunting. A transudate of serum protein enters the

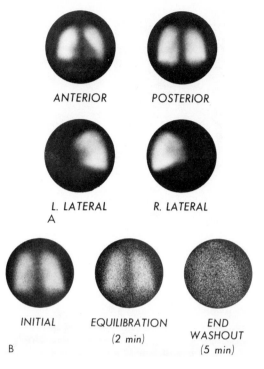

ANTERIOR   POSTERIOR

L. LATERAL   R. LATERAL

A

INITIAL   EQUILIBRATION   END
     (2 min)   WASHOUT

B   (5 min)

Fig. 4-1. (A) Normal four-view ^{99m}Tc-macroaggregated albumin perfusion lung scintiphoto study. Patient is 19-year-old girl evaluated for sickle cell lung disease. Note absence of perfusion in area occupied by cardiac silhouette, most prominent in anterior view. (B) Normal ^{133}Xe gas ventilation lung scintiphoto study in same patient. Patient was studied in posterior position.

alveolar ducts and becomes organized into a shiny eosinophilic substance which is the membrane of hyaline membrane disease. Disturbances of ventilation and perfusion as well as diffusion are prominent. In those infants who survive, recovery usually occurs by the first week of life. Since improved therapy has increased infant survival at younger gestational ages, more residual fibrosis and scarring of the lung are now reported. These residual abnormalities are referred to as "bronchopulmonary dysplasia," and are associated with disturbances in ventilation and perfusion, which are readily detected by radionuclide studies.

Illustrative case. This 1-month-old infant was born 7 weeks prematurely with hyaline membrane disease, which responded to treatment. The initial chest roentgenogram was compatible with this diagnosis but was nearly normal at the time of the radionuclidic study (Fig. 4-2).

Illustrative case. This 8-month-old infant was born 6–7 weeks prematurely with respiratory distress. His chest roentgenogram was initially compatible with hyaline membrane disease but was normal 1 month later. Subsequently he had two episodes of pneumonia presumably viral

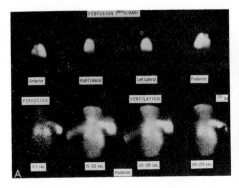
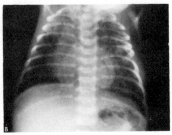

Fig. 4-2. Hyaline membrane disease. (A) Upper row, ^{99m}Tc-MAA (left to right; ant, rt lat, left lat, posterior view). Bottom row, ^{133}Xe, i.v. (left to right; 0–5 sec, 75–135 sec, 135–195 sec, 195–255 sec) post. There is generalized decrease in perfusion to right lung with focal defect in upper lobe. Xenon-133 does not enter right upper lobe after injection and is slow to washout from both lungs. Some ^{133}Xe persists in the veins of right arm, site of injection. (B) Roentgenogram.

in etiology. The associated roentgenographic infiltrates in both upper and middle lobes had resolved by the day of the scintiphoto study (Fig. 4-3).

Congenital lobar emphysema. As the name implies, hyperexpansion of one or more lobes of the lung occurs; compression atelectasis is usually seen in the remaining part of the lung. Although the emphysema is usually considered to result from some defect of the lung cartilage, it may also

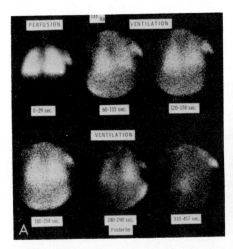
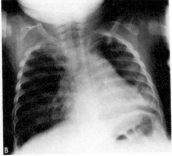

Fig. 4-3. Hyaline membrane disease. (A) ^{133}Xe, i.v. (0–29 sec, 60–113 sec, 120–174 sec, 180–234 sec, 240–290 sec, 310–457 sec) posterior view. Scintiphoto study is abnormal with mild generalized impairment of perfusion to left lung and mild impairment of ventilation evident from retention of radioactivity in both lungs. Last image reveals radioactivity in stomach which is due to air-swallowing. (B) Roentgenogram on same day.

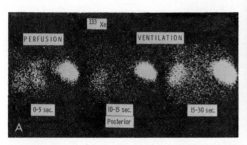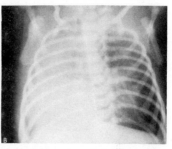

Fig. 4-4. Congenital lobar emphysema. (A) Scintiphoto study (posterior view) in patient was performed by injecting ^{133}Xe gas and observing its washout. First image (0–5 sec) reveals impairment of perfusion of left lung. Subsequent images at 10–15 sec and 15–30 sec indicate little ventilatory clearance from lung, consistent with lobar emphysema. (B) Roentgenogram.

result from aspirated foreign material, infection, or extraluminal compression due to mediastinal masses or bronchogenic cysts. Bronchial obstruction allows entry of air on inspiration but does not permit air to escape on expiration (9). Roentgenography shows hyperlucency, and displacement of the remaining lung and mediastinum may be present. Scintiphoto studies add information on the condition of the remaining lung tissue and the integrity of the bronchovascular system to the involved lung. This information may affect the management of the patient.

Illustrative case. This infant had cough, wheezing, dyspnea, progressive mediastinal displacement, and cyanosis resulting from the "ball-valve" type of obstruction of the involved lobe (Fig. 4-4).

Illustrative case. During the first few months of life, this 14-year-old boy had a severe, prolonged viral infection. Following a tonsillectomy at 11 years of age, he may have swallowed his vomitus. Neither of these events left him with any symptoms, and he was an active athlete. Examination of his chest revealed abnormalities over the left upper lung. Roentgenography and scintigraphy revealed abnormalities in the left upper lobe of the lung. The remainder of the lungs were normal. The latter information was of particular importance in the decision to surgically remove the bulla (Fig. 4-5).

Bacterial pneumonia. Intrauterine bacterial pneumonia is almost always associated with rupture of the amniotic membranes for a period longer than 24 hr and aspiration of septic material. The infant and child are also very susceptible to pneumonia. Intraluminal inflammatory reaction with accumulation of fluid and increase in total lung volume usually occurs. One or both lungs may be involved. The reduction in ventilation of the affected part of the lung is accompanied by a decrease in perfusion to the area (10); this may clinically mimic occlusion of the pulmonary artery.

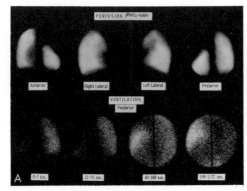
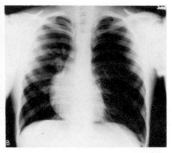

Fig. 4-5. Bullous emphysema. **(A)** Top row, ^{99m}Tc-MAA (as in Fig. 4-2). Bottom row, ^{133}Xe (0–7 sec, 22–55 sec, 55–388 sec, 398–1172 sec) posterior view. Scintiphoto studies reveal markedly reduced perfusion and ventilation to left upper lobe. During washout retention of ^{133}Xe in bulla and lung tissue adjacent to bulla, probably secondary to compression, is apparent. **(B)** Chest roentgenogram reveals hyperlucency of left upper lung and displacement of mediastinal structures into right hemithorax.

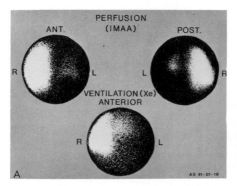
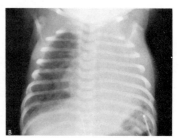

Fig. 4-6. Bacterial pneumonia. **(A)** There is extensive impairment of blood flow and ventilation to left lung. **(B)** Roentgenogram.

Illustrative case. This premature neonate was doing well despite losing 2 lb of weight since birth. Six weeks after birth the neonate suddenly became cyanotic and had a decreased blood oxygen tension. The chest roentgenogram revealed dense opacification of the left lung. The neonate had a low-grade fever and was presumed to have pneumonia. He was treated with an antibiotic without a favorable response. This caused concern that the infant may have become dehydrated and had a pulmonary thrombosis. Scintiphoto studies were requested to assist with the differential diagnosis (Fig. 4-6). Based on the results of this study, a primary ventilatory abnormality, such as pneumonia, was more likely than pulmonary vascular occlusive disease. The antibiotic regimen was modified, and the pneumonia responded. A few months later the child had a normal chest roentgenogram.

Bronchiolitis. Acute bronchiolitis is seen primarily in children under 18 months of age and is commonly believed to be due to the respiratory syncytial virus. It is associated with bronchiolar wall edema and cellular infiltrate. The lumen becomes obstructed with mucous and cellular debris, and air trapping with peripheral hyperexpansion results. This condition is a common cause of respiratory insufficiency and death in infants and young children. Those who recover often have residual lower airway obstruction and emphysema.

Illustrative case. This 4-year-old boy had experienced a severe upper respiratory infection at the age of 6 months but had recovered except for mild dyspnea on exertion and cough. The chest roentgenogram was not strikingly abnormal but demonstrated some decrease in vascular markings particularly in the lower portion of the right lung. The extent of ventilation and perfusion abnormalities present in this child's lungs were striking in view of his limited symptomatology and roentgenographic abnormalities (Fig. 4-7).

Pulmonary vascular occlusion. Although pulmonary embolism is a significant cause of adult morbidity and mortality, the condition is not as common in children. However, spontaneous thrombosis of pulmonary vessels is common in the neonate and infant and results in similar manifestations. Characteristically and commonly scintigraphy reveals perfusion abnormalities without remarkable ventilation abnormalities. This combination (also called increased V/Q ratio) is quite specific for pulmonary vascular occlusion, whereas diseases such as pneumonia, emphysema, and asthma produce ventilatory abnormalities as well as perfusion defects (*8, 10*). The chest roentgenogram frequently reveals no evidence of an infiltrate, a circumstance commonly encountered in embolism before or without infarction.

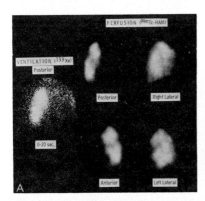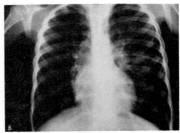

Fig. 4-7. Bronchiolitis. (A) Right, ^{99m}Tc-MAA. Upper row, posterior and right lateral. Lower row, anterior and left lateral. Marked decrease in perfusion throughout right lung is noted on perfusion scan as well as localized abnormalities on left. Following inhalation of ^{133}Xe gas (posterior view) severely impaired ventilation of right lung is apparent (left). (B) Roentgenogram.

Illustrative case. This 15-year-old girl was hospitalized because of ulcerative colitis. She developed clinical evidence of thrombophlebitis, and 3 days later had right pleuritic chest pain and hemoptysis. Diagnostic studies confirmed the presence of pulmonary emboli (Fig. 4-8).

Cystic fibrosis. Cystic fibrosis involves multiple organs, and pulmonary disease, while variable, is common and may be severe. Since the initial pulmonary lesion is in distal small airways, early changes may not be obvious clinically, roentgenographically, or by standard pulmonary function testing. Ventilation and perfusion scintigraphy have been suggested to be useful (*11, 12*).

Illustrative case. This 4-year-old child has cystic fibrosis, with abnormalities on the chest roentgenogram (Fig. 4-9).

Comments

At present no simple statement can be made relative to the role of radionuclidic lung studies in the pediatric population. It is safe to assume

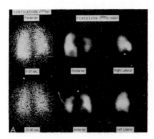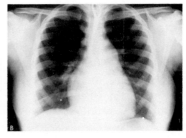

Fig. 4-8. Pulmonary embolism. (A) Right, perfusion study demonstrates two or more large defects in right lung and smaller perfusion defect at left base. Left, by contrast ^{133}Xe ventilation is relatively normal. (B) Chest roentgenogram is normal.

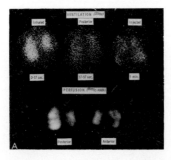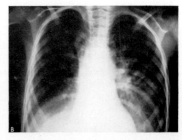

Fig. 4-9. Cystic fibrosis. (A) After injection of radioactive ^{99m}Tc-MAA particles severe impairment of perfusion within right lung, and several defects on left are apparent (bottom row: posterior, anterior). Upper row (posterior view): following inhalation of ^{133}Xe gas and breath-holding, marked general impairment of ventilation to right lung is evident as well as smaller, focal abnormalities in both lungs (0–17 sec, inhaled 37–57 sec). During washout of injected [133]Xe (5 min) there is uneven clearance and gas trapping in both lungs. (B) Roentgenogram.

that they will be used with increasing frequency for research and clinical applications because of their sensitivity and ready applicability to the pediatric patient. Methods comparable to those used in adults can be used in children older than 4 years (8). In younger children, however, a single injection of ^{133}Xe in solution provides an index of both regional perfusion and ventilation which is easier to accomplish. This method is particularly valuable in infants and neonates because it is rapid, requires no patient cooperation, results in a very low radiation dose, and can be repeated in serial studies. Radionuclidic studies of ventilation and perfusion can be performed in almost all children if the pediatrician and the nuclear medicine specialist have motivation and ingenuity.

Spontaneous pulmonary vascular occlusive disease which occurs in infants and pulmonary emboli in children are easily detected using radionuclides (8, 10). The pathophysiologic defects of pulmonary agenesis, bronchopulmonary sequestration, and foreign body aspiration may be demonstrated by these techniques. These techniques also appear to be useful in following patients with bronchial asthma, cystic fibrosis, congenital emphysema, and postinfection pulmonary abnormalities (1, 2, 11, 12). They are useful in children in whom pulmonary surgery is contemplated because they provide information on the type, location, and extent of disease and can be used to pre-operatively assess the likelihood of success of the operation, and postoperatively, the results. In hyaline membrane disease and other respiratory problems of the neonate, abnormal radionuclidic lung function studies have been observed in the face of a normal chest roentgenogram, particularly late in the course of the illness. The clinical implications of these observations are not yet established.

Although it is too early to establish the exact role of these studies in the practical management of pediatric pulmonary disease, there is reason to expect a substantial role for them. An understanding of this role and proper use of these techniques in children will require further collaboration between the pediatrician and the nuclear medicine specialist.

Acknowledgment

This work was supported in part by a Program Project Grant from NICHD, HD-04335.

References

1. PENDARVIS BC, SWISCHUK LE: Lung scanning in the assessment of respiratory disease in children. Am J Roentgenol Radium Ther Nucl Med 57: 313–321, 1969

2. ROBINSON AR, GOODRICH JK, SPOCK A: Inhalation and perfusion radionuclide studies of pediatric chest disease. Radiology 93: 1123–1128, 1969

3. TONG ECK, LIU L, POTTER RT, et al: Macro-aggregated RISA lung scan in congenital heart disease. Radiology 106: 585–592, 1973

4. DeNardo GL, Brody JS, Leach PJ, et al: Comparison of the pulmonary distribution of xenon-133 solution and iodine-131 macroaggregated albumin. *J Nucl Med* 8: 344, 1967

5. Shibel EM, Landis GA, Moser KM: Inhalation lung scanning evaluation radioaerosol versus radioxenon techniques. *Diseases of the Chest* 56: 284–289, 1969

6. Lopez-Majano V, Chernick V, Wagner HN, et al: Comparison of radio-isotope scanning and differential oxygen uptake of the lungs. *Radiology* 83: 697–698, 1964

7. Burdine JA, Murphy PH, Alagarsamy V, et al: Functional pulmonary imaging. *J Nucl Med* 13: 933–938, 1972

8. DeNardo GL, Goodwin DA, Ravasini R, et al: The ventilatory lung scan in the diagnosis of pulmonary embolism. *N Engl J Med* 282: 1334–1336, 1970

9. Fallat RJ, Powell MR, Kueppers F, et al: ^{133}Xe ventilatory studies in α_1 antitrypsin deficiency. *J Nucl Med* 14: 5–13, 1973

10. Sutherland JD, DeNardo GL, Brown DW: Lung scans with ^{131}I labeled macroaggregated human serum albumin (MAA). *Am J Roentgenol Radium Ther Nucl Med* 48: 416–426, 1966

11. Gyepes MT, Bennett LR, Hassakis PC: Regional pulmonary blood flow in cystic fibrosis. *Am J Roentgenol Radium Ther Nucl Med* 56: 567–575, 1969

12. Lamarre A, Reilly BJ, Bryan AC, et al: Early detection of pulmonary function abnormalities in cystic fibrosis. *Pediatrics* 50: 291–298, 1972

Chapter 5

Cardiovascular:
Radioisotopic Angiocardiography

Joseph P. Kriss

R adioisotopic angiocardiography, performed after the intravenous injection of ^{99m}Tc-labeled pertechnetate or albumin, is a simple, rapid,
and safe procedure which permits identification and physiologic assessment of a wide variety of congenital and acquired cardiovascular lesions.
These include atrial and ventricular septal defect, tetralogy of Fallot,
pulmonic stenosis, aortopulmonary window, transposition of the great
vessels, valvular stenosis and/or insufficiency, myocardial lesions, and
lesions of the great vessels. The simplicity of the procedure lends itself
to repeated measurements to assess the effects of therapy or to follow the
course of the disease.

A wide spectrum of congenital and acquired cardiovascular diseases have been studied which have particular application to the pediatric
age group (1–12).

Methods

Instrumentation. We have used the variable time-lapse videoscintiscope (VTV) for recording and selective playback of radioisotopic data
in most of our studies (13). Using this system one obtains analog images
of high quality especially suitable for qualitative analysis. The essential
feature of the instrument is the ability to play back and photograph any
portion of a recorded study any time after the injection of the radiopharmaceutical. The segment studied may be as short as $\frac{1}{60}$ sec to as long

as several minutes. This flexibility is important in obtaining the best images for qualitative analysis. The system also permits one to obtain double exposures of different portions of the records, e.g., right-sided and left-sided cardiac phases, a technique which is often useful in delineating anatomic relationships between different regions of the heart.

The addition of an on-line digital computer* permits most of the above-described functions to be carried out together with rapid computer analysis of isotopic data for quantitative evaluations. In general, the quality of the computer-processed images is not as good as that obtained with analog devices; however, this disadvantage is usually not crucial and is more than offset by the advantage of a quantitative capability.

Positioning technique. Adults and older children are usually studied in the sitting position. The detecting head of the Anger scintillation camera is positioned close over the precordium. Most often, two serial studies are carried out a few minutes apart. The first is in the nonrotated anterior position. However, this view is suboptimal for visualization of the region of the left atrium because of overlying heart structures. A better delineation of the left atrial chamber can be accomplished by centering the detector head over the left anterior axillary line in the left anterior oblique (LAO) position with the face of the detector directed downward at an angle of about 30 deg. This "modified LAO" view permits visualization of the left atrium free of overlying cardiac structures. In the absence of malrotation of the heart or marked right heart enlargement, the interventricular septum is commonly seen end-on in this view, providing separation of the left and right ventricular chambers. This view is of value for assessment of chamber size and myocardial wall thickness.

Infants and very young children are usually studied in the supine rather than the seated position, and the injection is made with the arm abducted. Special problems exist with young children. Venipuncture is more difficult. Crying is inevitable in the unsedated child, and the resulting involuntary Valsalva maneuver may interfere with bolus transit. The circulation times tend to be very rapid, and the size of the heart and the resulting scintiphoto image are very small. It is important, particularly in the assessment of septal defects, that the bolus enter the heart over a 1–2-sec interval. The prior injection of a sedative, use of small injection volume, and the use of an inlying venous catheter are valuable maneuvers to ensure prompt entry of the bolus. Scintiphoto image size in very young children or infants may be increased by substituting a pinhole collimator for the multichannel collimator usually used and positioning it close over the precordial area.

---

* Hewlett-Packard 5407A scintigraphic data analyzer.

Findings in Typical Clinical Situations

Normal. Figure 5-1 shows the angiographic findings typical of the normal adult subject studied in the anterior position. Usually the flow of radioactivity from the superior vena cava through the right atrium and right ventricle to the pulmonary artery lasts less than 8 sec and describes a typical U-shaped pattern. During the time of pulmonary transit of radioactivity there is little intracardiac activity for a few seconds when there has been a satisfactory bolus injection. Left atrial and left ventricular filling is commonly noted by 8–15 sec. These transit times are considerably shorter in children. However, the left atrium is not normally well visualized in the anterior view because of superimposed or adjacent activity in the left ventricular outflow tract and ascending aorta. The modified LAO view throws other cardiac and extracardiac structures off the left atrium for optimal visualization. Typically the arching course of the left pulmonary artery acts as a landmark, for the left atrium subsequently fills just beneath it.

Atrial septal defect (ASD). The scintiphotographic criteria of left-to-right intracardiac shunt at the atrial level stem from the fact that the radioactive blood, once it enters the left atrium on its first pass through the heart, in part is diverted through the septal defect and reappears in the right atrium, thereby initiating a continuous, recycling process. Thus in atrial-septal defect all four heart chambers and the lungs are concomitantly visualized. To make certain that the right atrium is clearly identified, the angiography study should be performed in both anterior and oblique positions. A typical study is shown in Fig. 5-2.

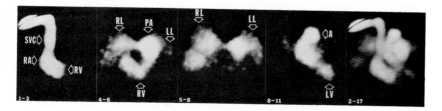

Fig. 5-1. Normal radionuclide angiocardiogram, anterior view. In this and subsequent figures, time interval (in seconds after injection) is shown for each scintiphotogram. Following abbreviations pertain in this and subsequent figures: SVC, superior vena cava; RA, right atrium; RV, right ventricle; PA, pulmonary artery; RL, right lung; LL, left lung; LA, left atrium; LV, left ventricle; A, aorta. Phase of right heart filling is seen in first frame. In second frame right ventricle, pulmonary artery, and initial lung activity is noted. Lung activity appears most clearly in Frame 3. Levo phase delineating left ventricle and ascending aorta is noted between 8 and 11 sec in Frame 4. Composite playthrough cardiopulmonary circulation phase from 2 through 17 sec is pictured in Frame 5.

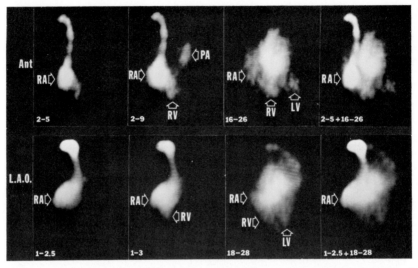

Fig. 5-2. Atrial septal defect, anterior and oblique positions. Note prominence of RA, "smudge" pattern in later phases (Frame 3) with activity present in RA (proved by double exposures, Frame 4) and other three heart chambers, failure to isolate on LV-aortic pattern and prolonged visualization of intracardiac activity. Pulmonary/systemic flow ratio was 1.6.

In ASD the following scintiphotographic findings may be noted:

1. Enlargement of the right atrium.
2. Loss of apparent intensity of bolus during initial cardiac filling phase as it passes from right atrium to right ventricle. (This sign is especially noted in the presence of large shunts and is probably due to dilution of the bolus by unlabeled blood entering the atrium across the septal defect.)
3. Enlargement of the pulmonary conus.
4. Persistent visualization of activity in all four cardiac chambers and lungs after first passage of bolus into lungs, tending to produce a long-lasting "smudge" pattern. This is the most characteristic and universal diagnostic angiographic feature of this lesion. It is important to document that the right atrium specifically contains radioactivity at all time phases of the study.
5. Relatively poor delineation of the aorta due to activity simultaneously present in the lungs.

The outstanding diagnostic angiographic features in the successfully operated patient are the prompt disappearance of the "smudge" pattern, normal right atrial emptying, and the ready visualization of an isolated left ventricular-aortic phase with a normal circulation time. However, right atrial enlargement and prominence of the pulmonary conus region may persist, at least for several weeks.

Our results indicate a high sensitivity of the method with respect to shunt magnitude. Shunts associated with a calculated pulmonary/systemic flow ratio of only 1.2:1 have been readily visualized. The largest shunt was associated with a pulmonary/systemic flow ratio of 3:1.

Ventricular septal defect (VSD). The recycling of blood from left ventricle back into right ventricle following initial filling of the former chamber results in a characteristic abnormal angiographic pattern resembling but not identical to that of atrial septal defect (Fig. 5-3). The noteworthy diagnostic features of VSD are:

1. Persistent visualization of the right ventricle, lungs, left atrium, and left ventricle, but not the right atrium after first passage of the bolus through the right heart and lungs.
2. Relatively poor delineation of the aorta due to activity simultaneously present in the lungs.

The demonstration that, during recycling, the right atrium is not refilling serves to distinguish VSD from ASD. The smallest ventricular shunt demonstrated by the radioisotopic test was associated with a pulmonary/systemic flow ratio of 1.2:1.

Tetralogy of Fallot. In patients with tetralogy of Fallot, we have demonstrated a variety of abnormalities, depending to some extent on the age of the patient and whether or not previous cardiac surgery had been performed. Figure 5-4 gives the following findings in a previously untreated adult:

1. Markedly diminished caliber of pulmonary outflow tract and main pulmonary branches due to pulmonary artery atresia.
2. Early appearance of activity in left ventricle immediately after right ventricular filling due to right-to-left shunt across a ventricular septal defect.

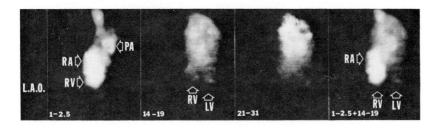

Fig. 5-3. Ventricular septal defect, oblique position. Note "smudge" patterns in late phases (Frames 2 and 3), late visualization of RV and L, but not RA (compare Frames 2 and 4), and prolonged visualization of cardiopulmonary activity. Pulmonic/systemic flow ratio was 1.2.

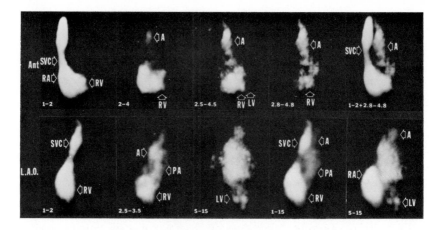

Fig. 5-4. Tetralogy of Fallot, anterior position (top row) and oblique position (bottom row). In anterior note very early filling of aorta (A), Frames 2–4, directly from RV (Frame 4) but no visualization of pulmonic outflow tract. LV also was faintly visualized early in original scintiphoto (Frame 3). In oblique study both PA and A are visualized early (Frame 2), and LV was not seen until later (Frame 3). Intense activity above LV (Frame 3) was due to abnormal bronchial arterial channels, demonstrated more definitively by roentgenographic studies.

3. Early filling of the aorta immediately after right ventricular filling due to right over-riding of the aorta on the right ventricular chamber.

Aortopulmonary window. A variable right-to-left shunt between the main pulmonary artery and the ascending aorta was demonstrated in one patient who developed striking cyanosis and poor exercise tolerance on slight exertion but who was minimally cyanotic at rest. Radioisotopic angiocardiography was performed before and after exercise. Both studies were abnormal (Fig. 5-5). The scintigraphic study was unique and revealed the following findings:

1. Asymmetrical main pulmonary trunk with anomalous right-sided tract leading to the region of the ascending aorta.
2. Demonstration of activity in ascending aorta and arch nearly synchronous with presence of maximal pulmonary artery activity and before delineation of left ventricle.
3. Rapid loss of radioactivity from the heart immediately after delineating the right-sided cardiac phase.

The findings are similar to those expected in patent ductus arteriosus with Eisenmenger physiology except that in the latter the descending rather than the ascending aorta would be visualized, and a ductus involving the right side of the pulmonary trunk would be unusual.

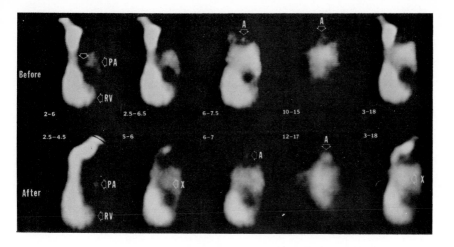

Fig. 5-5. Aortopulmonary window, anterior position. Note asymmetry of PA to right, with tract filling ascending aortic area (Frames 1 and 2, top arrow), early aortic activity (Frame 3). Top row before exercise, bottom row after exercise.

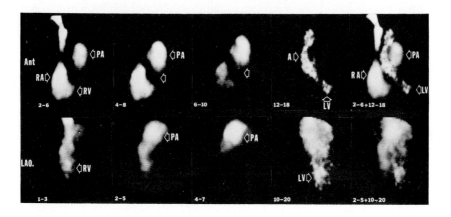

Fig. 5-6. Pulmonic stenosis, anterior and oblique positions. Anteriorly note relatively small-sized cavity of RV (Frames 1 and 2), persistent narrowing in right ventricular outflow tract due to hypertrophied infundibulum (arrow, Frames 2, 3), persistent filling of dilated main pulmonary artery (PA) just beyond narrowing, and delayed filling of LV and aorta. In oblique position, note RV cavity is relatively small, PA is dilated and retains activity over long interval (Frames 2, 3).

Pulmonic stenosis. Figure 5-6 shows the marked abnormalities seen in a patient with severe pulmonic valvular stenosis:

1. Prolonged residence of the bolus in the right side of the heart.
2. Persistent and striking narrowing of the pulmonic valve area.

3. Marked post-stenotic dilatation of the pulmonary trunk.
4. Relatively small-size cavity of the right ventricle due to right ventricular hypertrophy.

Transposition of the great vessels. Figure 5-7 shows strikingly abnormal findings in an adult patient with transposition of the great vessels and pulmonic stenosis:

1. Early filling of aorta immediately after filling of right ventricle.
2. Early marked loss of cardiac activity.
3. Very faint visualization of left ventricle and pulmonary artery, so that right heart and aorta were the only portions of the heart well seen.
4. Visualization of a small, poorly functioning Blalock anastomosis which had been made earlier.

The findings bear some resemblance to those seen in tetralogy of Fallot, as might be expected since the physiology of transposition with pulmonic stenosis is similar to that of tetralogy.

Figure 5-8 shows a postoperative scintiphotographic sequence in a cyanotic 13-year-old child who had undergone a successful Mustard

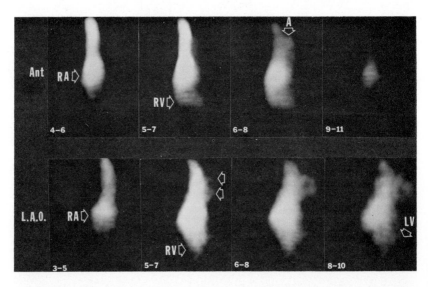

Fig. 5-7. Transposition of great vessels, anterior and oblique positions. Anteriorly note very early filling of aorta A (Frames 2, 3), rapid disappearance of cardiac activity (Frame 4), failure to visualize left ventricle or pulmonary artery. In oblique position note filling of two outflow tracts after RV filling (arrows, Frames 2 and 3) corresponding to aorta and pulmonary artery joined by Blalock anastomosis (Frame 3); LV is only faintly visualized (Frame 4).

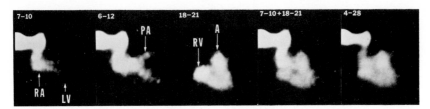

Fig. 5-8. Transposition of great vessels, anterior position, 1 week postoperatively (Mustard procedure). Note filling of LV from upper part of RA (Frame 1), subsequent filling of PA (Frame 2), later filling of RV and A (Frame 3). Identity of chambers is proven by comparing composite (Frame 4) with previous frames.

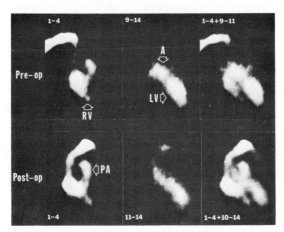

Fig. 5-9. Supravalvular aortic stenosis, anterior position, pre- and postoperatively (1 week). Preoperatively note sharp cutoff of activity just above aortic root (A) at point of stenosis and failure to visualize ascending aorta (Frame 2), LV dilatation. Postoperatively note normal aortic filling (Frame 2), slightly smaller LV.

procedure for transposition of the great arteries 1 week earlier. As a consequence of her malformation, unoxygenated blood entered the aorta from the right ventricle while blood exited the left ventricle via the pulmonary artery; a large ventricular septal defect was present also. The surgical procedure involved closure of the ventricular defects, diversion of right atrial blood to left ventricle, and left atrial blood to right ventricle, thereby establishing a physiologically normal circulation.

Supravalvular aortic stenosis. Unusual findings were demonstrated in an 11-year-old boy with a murmur suggesting aortic stenosis (Fig. 5-9). However, other diagnostic tests, as well as radioisotopic angiocardiography, indicated that the stenosis of the aorta was supravalvular. One week after surgical correction of the lesion, radioisotopic angiography demonstrated marked improvement in aortic filling.

Coarctation of aorta. Lesions of the arch or descending aorta are usually best studied in the left anterior oblique position. The author urges caution in interpretation of narrowing of the descending aorta, however, since the descending aorta normally may appear to diminish in caliber just beyond the arch. This finding is partly due to anatomic change in caliber of the aorta and partly due to the greater distance (and therefore diminished scintigraphic intensity) of the lower aorta from the detector. It is essential that an abrupt change in aorta size and contour be demonstrated before a diagnosis of coarctation can be made.

Discussion

Our results of intravenous radioisotopic angiocardiography demonstrate that markedly abnormal and distinguishable scintiphotographic patterns are obtained in a variety of specific cardiovascular diseases. The conditions include congenital and acquired heart disease, involving both right- and left-sided lesions, and diseases of the great vessels and pericardium. In many respects intravenous radioisotopic angiocardiography resembles forward angiography performed by intravenous injection of contrast material. Advances in our knowledge of congenital heart disease permit us to interpret the dynamic scintiphotographs as representations of normal or deranged physiologic events. Combined with an understanding of pathologic congenital cardiac anatomy, this relatively simple, noninvasive, speedy, and safe technique becomes an attractive and useful clinical procedure with wide applicability.

The findings we have enumerated for specific lesions have been a reasonably good guide to diagnosis. With experience, we have come to recognize that each pattern represents a physiological circumstance (e.g., left-to-right shunt or obstruction to pulmonary flow), which when correlated with the apparent anatomy suggests a given cardiac lesion. We recognize that different anatomic abnormalities may give similar physiologic syndromes and may be very difficult to distinguish by this technique. For example, tetralogy of Fallot, double outlet right ventricle, transposition of the great vessels with pulmonic stenosis, and ventricular septal defect with pulmonary hypertension form an incomplete list of lesions which might be expected to give similar scintiphotograms with the intravenous technique we have described. Nevertheless, as a screening procedure and for serial study of the effects of medical or surgical intervention the intravenous radioisotopic angiocardiogram provides physiologic and anatomic information not readily obtainable by other noninvasive techniques.

The atraumatic nature of this examination deserves special emphasis in the pediatric age group. This procedure can easily be performed on an outpatient, and therefore removes from the physician the psychological burdens associated with hospitalization of a child who is otherwise doing well.

In general, we recommend that radioisotopic angiocardiography be performed as a screening procedure prior to cardiac catheterization or selective contrast angiography.

The sensitivity of the method, especially in the assessment of septal defects, is excellent, e.g., capable of indicating the presence of left-to-right shunts associated with a pulmonary artery-to-systemic flow ratio of only 1.2:1. The procedure has been especially helpful in ruling out recurrence of shunts in surgically treated patients with persistent or developing cardiac murmurs.

Acknowledgment

Figure 5-1 is reprinted from *Semin Nucl Med 3:* 177–190, 1973. Figure 5-2 is reprinted from *Radiol Clin North Am* 9: 369–383, 1971. Figure 5-3 to 5-9 are reprinted from *J Nucl Med 13,* 31–40, 1972. All are reprinted with permission of the publisher.

References

1. KRISS JP: Diagnosis of pericardial effusion by radioisotopic angiocardiography. *J Nucl Med* 10: 233–241, 1969

2. KRISS JP, MATIN P: Diagnosis of congenital and acquired cardiovascular diseases by radioisotopic angiocardiography. *Trans Assoc Am Physicians* 82: 109–119, 1970

3. MATIN P, KRISS JP: Radioisotopic angiocardiography: findings in mitral stenosis and mitral insufficiency. *J Nucl Med* 11: 723–730, 1970

4. MATIN P, RAY G, KRISS JP: Combined superior vena cava obstruction and pericardial effusion demonstrated by radioisotopic angiocardiography. *J Nucl Med* 11: 78–80, 1970

5. KRISS JP, ENRIGHT LP, HAYDEN WG, et al: Radioisotopic angiocardiography: wide scope of applicability in diagnosis and evaluation of therapy in diseases of the heart and great vessels. *Circulation* 43: 792–808, 1971

6. KRISS JP, FREEDMAN GS, ENRIGHT LP, et al: Radioisotopic angiocardiography: preoperative and postoperative evaluation of patients with diseases of the heart and aorta. *Radiol Clin North Am* 9: 369–383, 1971

7. KRISS JP, ENRIGHT LP, HAYDEN WT, et al: Radioisotopic angiocardiography: findings in congenital heart disease. *J Nucl Med* 13: 31–40, 1972

8. KERBER RE, GREENE RA, COHN LH, et al: Multiple left ventricular outflow obstructions—Aortic valvular and supravalvular stenosis and coarctation of the aorta. *J Thorac Cardiovasc Surg* 63: 374–379, 1972

9. KERBER RE, RIDGES JD, KRISS JP, et al: Unruptured aneurysm of the sinus of Valsalva producing right ventricular outflow obstruction. *Am J Med* 53: 775–783, 1972

10. MAXFIELD WS, MECKSTROTH GR: Technetium-99m superior vena cavography. *Radiology* 92: 913–917, 1969

11. DeLAND FH, FELMAN AH: Pericardial tumor compared with pericardial effusion. *J Nucl Med* 13: 697–698, 1972

12. BONTE FJ, CHRISTENSEN EE, CURRY TS: Tc^{99m} Pertechnetate angiocardiography in the diagnosis of superior mediastinal masses and pericardial effusions. *Am J Roentgenol Radium Ther Nucl Med* 107: 404–412, 1969

13. KRISS JP, BONNER WA, LEVINTHAL EC: Variable time-lapse videoscintiscope: a modification of the scintillation camera designed for rapid flow studies. *J Nucl Med* 10: 249–251, 1969

Chapter **6**

Cardiovascular: Shunt Quantitation

William L. Ashburn and Naomi P. Alazraki

A s we gain experience in radionuclide imaging with the gamma scintillation camera, new applications for the evaluation of specific diagnostic problems are suggested. In this regard, radionuclide angiography has achieved increasing prominence as a noninvasive method to assess a variety of cardiocirculatory disorders both in adults and in children. Since significant numbers of patients in the pediatric age group present a diagnostic problem of differentiating functional heart murmurs from congenital heart disease associated with a left-to-right shunt, pediatric cardiologists have expressed considerable interest in applying the current technologic advances in acquisition and processing of dynamic scintillation camera data to this problem.

Radionuclide angiography has been used in the study of altered cardiac dynamics in pediatric patients for nearly 5 years. There is a natural tendency to compare the quality of the serial radionuclide images of the heart with high-quality x-ray contrast angiocardiograms obtained at the time of cardiac catheterization. Wish as we might that radionuclide angiographic quality could approach radiographic quality with regard to the visualization of cardiac structures, we must recognize the fact that even the best radionuclide angiograms can demonstrate only the grossest changes in morphology and alterations in cardiac function. Thus one might question the necessity or desirability of performing this kind of examination when contrast angiography is undoubtedly better able to define anatomical features in the beating heart. The answer lies in our potential ability to derive quantitative information from the radionuclide studies, and in the extreme safety and the simplicity of the technique associated with relatively little radiation exposure. Indeed, the procedure entails nothing more arduous than an intravenous injection of a bolus of physiologically inert substance (^{99m}Tc-pertechnetate), followed by imaging with the commonly available scintillation camera. This permits the screening of certain outpatients without the initial requirement of cardiac catheterization and of those patients considered to be too ill to undergo the injection of radiographic contrast material.

A comparison between early examples (1, 2) of sequential cardiac scintiphotos obtained during the transit of a radioactive bolus through the cardiopulmonary circulation with the striking images shown in Chapter 5 clearly indicates that significant advances have taken place in instrumentation and technique during the past several years. While those of us who are experienced in reviewing these studies appreciate that a great many acquired and congenital abnormalities can be recognized (3, 4), we know that precise *quantitation* of the altered circulatory dynamics requires analysis of the time-dependent counting-rate data derived from specific anatomic regions of interest (e.g., cardiac chambers, lung fields) during the intracardiac transit of the injected bolus.

Before proceeding with specific examples relating to the detection and quantitation of left-to-right shunts, certain technical considerations require clarification.

Method of Injection

It is sometimes possible to obtain acceptable radionuclide angiograms following the injection into a peripheral vein of any volume of ^{99m}Tc-pertechnetate up to several milliliters. However, we have consistently found that a small volume (less than 0.5 ml) injected into either the external jugular or femoral vein followed by a flush of sterile saline results in decidedly better studies when quantitative data analysis is required. Furthermore, sedation of the child is advisable since it not only reduces the anxiety associated with the procedure but appears to improve the quality of the study. Crying and breath-holding tend to impede the transit of the radioactive bolus into the right atrium, thereby significantly altering the curves on which the quantitative data are based. We would caution against proceeding with the quantitative analysis of regional scintillation data unless these technical requirements are met.

In general, 200 μCi/kg (up to a maximum of 8 mCi) of ^{99m}Tc-pertechnetate is injected per study. Other chemical forms of ^{99m}Tc can be substituted for pertechnetate since after the first circulation through the heart and lungs rapid blood clearance of the radioactive agent is desirable. Thus ^{99m}Tc-sulfur colloid (cleared rapidly by the liver) or [99m]Tc-

DTPA (cleared rapidly by the kidneys) can be used. On the other hand, if blood volume or cardiac output determinations (with or without ejection fraction) are to be performed, ^{99m}Tc-human serum albumin (cleared slowly from the blood) is the agent of choice.

Imaging and Data Analysis

In Chapter 5 the importance of scintillation camera detector position with respect to the heart is discussed. The anterior projection is convenient and is usually satisfactory for a general appraisal of the cardiopulmonary anatomy and for specific analysis of the counting-rate "dilution" curves derived from both lung fields. The left anterior oblique projection modified by angulation of the detector toward the feet provides better separation of the cardiac chambers but is associated with a poorer view of both lung fields.

Radionuclide angiocardiography in infants and small children presents additional technical difficulties because of the relatively small size of the heart and lungs. Since the inherent resolution of the scintillation camera detector is fixed, maneuvers to "magnify" the heart and lungs to the full available view of the detector are desirable and can be best accomplished by using a "converging" low-energy collimator with which maximum sensitivity and resolution at depth are preserved.

To adequately evaluate the counting-rate "dilution curves" (or "time-activity histograms") derived from specific regions of anatomic interest, requires special equipment to record the raw scintillation camera positional data for subsequent playback and analysis. A variety of tape recording systems are commercially available for this purpose. The more sophisticated systems usually use a small digital computer which is a necessity for the more complex analyses of the immense amount of data accumulated during the recording period. Common to all of the systems is their ability to faithfully record at high data rates and to generate, upon replay, a facsimile of the original images for the identification of anatomy and placement of electronic boundaries commonly called "regions-of-interest" (ROIs). Multiple (up to 12 or 16) ROIs can be chosen and plots of time as a function of counting rate from each region made. The net result is essentially similar to placing separate carefully collimated scintillation probes over the chest area except that in the case of the scintillation camera the ROIs are chosen after review of the serial radionuclide images and can be electronically repositioned as often as necessary upon replay of the original tape recording.

Detection of Left-to-Right Shunts

During the past few years investigators in "nuclear cardiology" have been perfecting radionuclide methods of detecting and quantitating left-to-right and right-to-left shunts. Four approaches to the analysis of data obtained during radionuclide cardiopulmonary angiography for shunt detection are described in the following sections.

C2/C1 determination from pulmonary radionuclide dilution curves. The C2/C1 ratio for detection of left-to-right shunts was first reported in 1962 by Folse and Braunwald (5). These investigators described a technique for obtaining pulmonary vascular radionuclide dilution curves following the intravenous injection of ^{131}I-labeled diodrast, using a single-probe detector placed over a region of the patient's chest thought to represent peripheral lung vasculature. They used a strip-chart recorder to plot the appearance and disappearance of the radionuclide beneath the probe. The resulting curve represented the time-to-concentration relationship of the radionuclide passing through the pulmonary vascular bed beneath the probe and was somewhat analogous to indicator dilution dye curves obtained during cardiac catheterization.

According to this method two points on the curve are defined and measured: C1 and C2 (Fig. 6-1). C1 is the point of maximum counting rate and C2 is defined as a point on the curve which occurs at a time T2 following the point of maximum activity. T2 is equal to T1 which, in turn, is equal to the period of time between the earliest detection of radioactivity and the point of maximum activity. The ratio of C2/C1 is then expressed as a percentage. Figure 6-1 gives typical curves, showing that in patients with left-to-right shunts the ascending portion of the curve rises rapidly to a peak, but the descending limb of the curve is prolonged because of the recirculation of tracer through the left-to-right shunt and lungs. This results in a greater C2/C1 ratio than that expected in the normal.

Using the scintillation camera and imaging over the heart and lungs, we have examined a large series of both normals and patients with left-to-

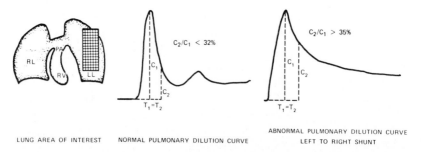

LUNG AREA OF INTEREST   NORMAL PULMONARY DILUTION CURVE

ABNORMAL PULMONARY DILUTION CURVE
LEFT TO RIGHT SHUNT

Fig. 6-1. Radionuclide dilution curves obtained from regions-of-interest corresponding to left lung in normal (center) and in patient with left-to-right shunt (right). Region-of-interest (grid overlying part of left lung) is generated electronically, but its position and size are controlled by physician upon replay of original data. C2/C1 values less than 32% are considered normal and values greater than 35% are compatible with left-to-right shunt. Percentages do not indicate degree of shunting.

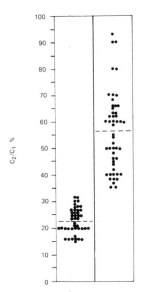

Fig. 6-2. C2/C1 values in 93 patients with and without left-to-right shunts. Values ranged from 15 to 32% in normals (column on left) and from 35 to 94% in patients with left-to-right shunt (column on right).

right shunts (6). Regions-of-interest were placed over one or both lung fields, carefully avoiding any portion of the heart or great vessels within the ROIs. With the aid of a computer, plots of counts appearing within the defined region against time were generated. C2/C1 ratios of less than 32% were consistently calculated in normals, while in patients with left-to-right shunt the C2/C1 ratios were greater than 35%.

Figure 6-2 shows the results of this study in 93 patients, nearly half of which underwent cardiac catheterization for confirmation of the presence or absence of a left-to-right shunt. The remaining patients were classified as having shunts or no shunts on the basis of clinical, radiographic, electrocardiographic, vector analysis, and phonocardiographic data. All patients ranged in aged from 2 days to 45 years. Ninety percent were under 18 years of age and half were under the age of 5. In patients with left-to-right shunts the range of C2/C1 ratios was 35–96% with an average value of 57%. Seven of the patients who underwent cardiac catheterization had trivial left-to-right shunt detected by hydrogen probe only. Even so, all of these patients had C2/C1 ratios of greater than 35%.

An attempt was made to quantitate the degree of left-to-right shunting by the C2/C1 method. Although there was some correlation between the C2/C1 ratios and the magnitude of the shunt, precise quantitation was not possible by this technique alone.

Rosenthall (7) has reported on a similar technique and determined C2/C1 values to be somewhat higher and more widely spread in normals than in our series. It is significant to note, however, that no attempt was made to inject the radioactive bolus as close to the heart as possible (i.e., femoral or jugular vein) as in our cases. It should be remembered that other conditions resulting in impaired right ventricular function can be associated with an abnormal C2/C1 ratio. However, when these can be excluded on clinical grounds, as in most cases in which this procedure might be helpful in the screening of shunt suspects, the C2/C1 determination would appear to have sufficient sensitivity to be of value.

Quantitative Qp/Qs determinations based on the pulmonary time-activity histogram. In an attempt to quantitate the severity of left-to-right shunting in children, Maltz and Treves (8) have suggested an ingenious method of pulmonary dilution curve analysis. A gamma variate is fit by computer to the ascending limb and first portion of the descending limb of the pulmonary dilution curve (Fig. 6-3). Based on this derived function, the remainder of the descending limb is extrapolated down to the baseline. The area under this curve corresponds to the counts obtained during the flow of the radioactive bolus through the lungs without accounting for recirculation through the left-to-right shunt. The extrapolated curve is then subtracted point for point from the original dilution curve resulting in a second curve. After application of a similar gamma variate fit to this curve, a third curve is derived, the area under which corresponds to the recirculation of the radioactivity through a left-to-right shunt and into the pulmonary ROI. The ratio of pulmonary blood flow (Qp) to system blood flow (Qs) is calculated according to the formula shown in Fig. 6-3. These investigators suggested that the Qp/Qs could be accurately quantitated when it fell between 1.2 and 3.0. A correlation coefficient of 0.91 was calculated when Qp/Qs values determined by oximetry were compared with the Qp/Qs determined by the radionuclide method in 25 patients.

Analysis of specific heart chamber radionuclide dilution curves. Bosnjakovic and associates (9) have reported on their experience in detecting both left-to-right and right-to-left shunts by observing the radionuclide dilution curves from selected ROIs corresponding to specific chambers of the heart. Their findings are summarized in Fig. 6-4 which shows theoretical curves which might be obtained from regions-of-interest over the right and left heart chambers during the passage of a bolus of ^{99m}Tc-sulfur colloid. In a normal patient there is a prompt rise to the peak height and a fall to the baseline activity when one monitors both the right or left heart chambers—the right heart peak, of course, appearing before the left heart peak. In right-to-left cardiac shunts a single peak is noted in the right heart curve, but an abnormal early peak, representing the blood radioactivity shunted through the defect from right to left, is detected simultaneously from the ROI corresponding to the left heart chamber. In left-to-right intracardiac shunts an abnormal late peak

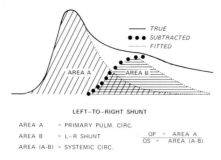

LEFT—TO—RIGHT SHUNT

AREA A	= PRIMARY PULM. CIRC.
AREA B	= L–R SHUNT
AREA (A-B)	= SYSTEMIC CIRC.

$$\frac{QP}{QS} = \frac{AREA\ A}{AREA\ (A-B)}$$

Fig. 6-3. Gamma variate fit method of Maltz and Treves (see text). Area A corresponds to that portion of radioactive bolus which passed through lung (i.e., Qp) before recirculation through same region of lung by left-to-right shunt. Derived Area B corresponds to shunted portion of radioactive bolus, while difference (Area A–Area B) represents net systemic output (i.e., Qs).

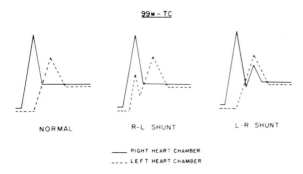

$^{99m}-TC$

NORMAL   R-L SHUNT   L-R SHUNT

_____ RIGHT HEART CHAMBER
_ _ _ _ LEFT HEART CHAMBER

Fig. 6-4. Peak appearance times of radioactive bolus in specific heart chambers as set by regions-of-interest (see text) can be used to detect both left-to-right and right-to-left shunts.

of activity is detected over the right heart, representing the shunted radio-active tracer from the left-to-right heart chambers. In theory, if precise placement of the ROIs could be made to correspond exclusively to the atria and/or ventricles, one could determine the probable site of shunting.

Analysis of right and left heart chamber time-activity histograms to determine Qp/Qs in intracardiac shunts. Weber, et al (10), using a small computer and the scintillation camera, have reported a method of detection and quantitation of left-to-right and right-to-left shunts by analyzing the dilution curves from specific cardiac chambers in a way quite similar to the technique used in quantitating the Qp/Qs proposed by Maltz and Treves (see above). As with the method of Bosnjakovic, et al described earlier, the accuracy of this method would appear to be only as good as one's ability to accurately identify and isolate specific heart chambers for the selection of the ROIs. Although only six left-to-right and two right-to-left shunt cases were analyzed in this fashion, these investigators suggested that their technique might be expected to provide reliable data in similar cases.

Summary

It is clear that the use of radionuclide techniques in left-to-right shunt detection is relatively new and that many more patients must be studied to accumulate a reliable experience with these methods in order to select the best approach. Even so, it appears that radionuclide methods may prove to be excellent screening procedures for patients with heart murmurs of undetermined etiology as well as a tool for following pre- and postoperative shunt patients. We would not presume that these techniques will in any way replace cardiac catheterizations for complete diagnostic evaluation but rather they may be used to indicate the need for this more definitive, but necessarily more expensive and traumatic, procedure.

References

1. MASON DT, ASHBURN WL, HARBERT JC, et al: Rapid visualization of the heart and great vessels in man using the wide-field Anger scintillation camera, radioisotope-angiography following the injection of technetium-99m. *Circulation* 39: 19–28, 1968

2. BURKE G, HALKO A, GOLDBERG D: Dynamic clinical studies with radio-isotopes and the scintillation camera. IV. ^{99m}Tc-sodium pertechnetate cardiac blood flow studies. *J Nucl Med* 10: 270–280, 1969

3. HAGAN AD, FRIEDMAN WF, ASHBURN WL, et al: Further applications of scintillation scanning techniques to the diagnosis and management of infants and children with congenital heart disease. *Circulation* 45: 858–867, 1972

4. HAYDEN WG, KRISS JP: Scintiphotographic studies of acquired cardiovascular disease. *Semin Nucl Med* 3: 177–190, 1973

5. FOLSE R, BRAUNWALD E: Pulmonary vascular dilution curves recorded by external detection in the diagnosis of left-to-right shunts. *Br Heart J* 24: 166–172, 1962

6. ALAZRAKI NP, ASHBURN WL, HAGAN AD, et al: Detection of left-to-right shunts with the scintillation camera pulmonary dilution curve. *J Nucl Med* 13: 142–147, 1972

7. ROSENTHALL L: Nucleographic screening of patients for left-to-right cardiac shunts. *Radiology* 99: 601–604, 1972

8. MALTZ DL, TREVES S: Quantitative radionuclide angiography: determination of Qp:Qs in children. *Circulation* 47: 1049–1056, 1973

9. BOSNJAKOVIC VB, BENNETT LR, GREENFIELD LD, et al: Dual isotope method for diagnosis of intracardiac shunts. *J Nucl Med* 14: 514–521, 1973

10. WEBER PM, DOS REMEDIOS LV, JASKO IA: Quantitative radioisotopic angiocardiography. *J Nucl Med* 13: 815–822, 1972

Chapter 7

Liver

Hirsch Handmaker

The widespread availability of radiopharmaceuticals that localize within the reticuloendothelial and hepatobiliary systems has been of great value in assessing the functional and anatomic status of the liver in both pediatric and adult patients. The improved radiobiological characteristics of newer agents, the ability to detect smaller abnormalities, and the capability of obtaining rapid serial images has specifically aided the young patient, and reduced the concern of the pediatrician through a more favorable risk: benefit ratio (1).

Choice of Radiopharmaceuticals

Colloidal preparations. The radionuclide preparations that contain submicron size particles are cleared from the bloodstream by phagocytic Küpffer cells of the liver's reticuloendothelial system and remain there until they are either metabolized or become "permanently" trapped. All liver-*imaging* nuclide preparations that are currently of clinical importance use the RES "trap", despite the fact that only 40% of the liver cell population and 10% of its mass is actually reticuloendothelial in nature. Various polygonal cell-specific radiopharmaceuticals have been investigated as liver-imaging agents including rose bengal (^{131}I-RB) and [99]Mo-molybdate (2), but their physical and biological characteristics have made them impractical. Technetium-99m-labeled-sulfur colloid has become the most popular agent, replacing the formerly used [198]Au-colloid. The ^{99m}Tc has several advantages over [198]Au, including more desirable

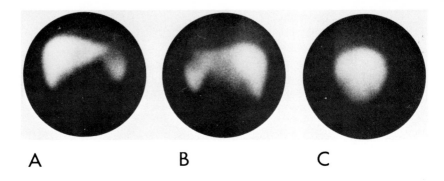

A   B   C

Fig. 7-1. Normal liver scintiphoto made with ^{99m}Tc-sulfur colloid.
(A) Anterior view; (B) posterior view; (C) right lateral view.

physical characteristics (i.e., lower energy, shorter half-life), factors of particular importance in pediatric patients. In addition, it is widely available and inexpensive. Radiation exposures are given in Table 8-3.

The normal ^{99m}Tc-sulfur colloid scintiphoto study is shown in Fig. 7-1. At least three views (anterior, posterior, and right lateral) are obtained in all patients.

^{131}**I-rose bengal.** One of the first radionuclides used in medical diagnosis was ^{131}I-RB. It is representative of the radiopharmaceuticals that actually localize within polygonal cells. These cells comprise 60% of liver cells and 90% of liver mass. Rose bengal is cleared from the blood by active transport across the hepatic polygonal cell membrane, excreted into the biliary passages, and ultimately into the gastrointestinal tract. No significant re-absorption occurs from the GI tract. It is important that in the presence of obstruction, ^{131}I-RB as well as dissociated ^{131}I is returned to the circulation and excreted by the kidneys.

Images made at 30 min–2 hr in *normal patients* show the pattern of polygonal cell uptake. Maximum uptake will occur at 20–30 min. Twenty five to 55 min after injection, a fall in hepatic activity occurs, and biliary and/or GI activity increases with filling in of the intrahepatic

---

TABLE 7-1. Correlation of ^{131}I-RB Retention with Liver Pathology*†

Greater than 86% = Extensive polygonal cell disease ("failure") with or without intestinal excretion
Less than 86% without intestinal excretion = complete extrahepatic obstruction
Less than 80% with excretion and uniform distribution = indeterminate etiology
60–86% = consistent with acute hepatitis and varying degrees of obstruction
Less than 60% = Normal.

---

* After Nordyke and Blahd (*4*).

† % retention $= \dfrac{20 \text{ min}}{5 \text{ min}}$ counts $\times$ 100.

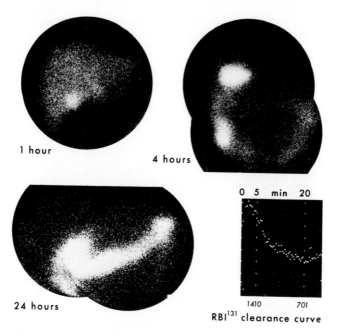

1 hour

4 hours

0 5   min   20

24 hours

1410   701

RBI[131] clearance curve

Fig. 7-2. Normal ^{131}I-RB excretion study. Note dense accumulation of material in gallbladder at 1 and 4 hr, small bowel accumulation at 4 hr, and radionuclide "colonogram" at 24 hr. ^{131}I-RB clearance curve indicates 50% clearance (5 min = 1,410 cpm, 20 min = 701 cpm).

biliary radicles. An outline can be seen of small or large bowel concentration of the radionuclide. The gallbladder will be visualized in most normal patients as well as in those with *distal* common duct obstructions.

Modifications have been made in the ^{131}I-RB studies to obtain maximum information. Since the dye is cleared from the blood exponentially after an equilibration time (about 5 min), its clearance can be used as a measure of liver function (3). Correlation with the clearance rates with various disease entities has been made (4) (Table 7-1). The clearance rate is determined by placing a probe or camera (scintillation detector) in conjunction with a scaler over a nonhepatic blood pool (i.e., the head), and counts are recorded for 30 min. The 5- and 20-min counts are used for the calculation of clearance. Scans and/or scintiphotos are then made over liver and abdomen. Figure 7-2 shows a normal rose bengal excretion study and curve.

Liver Imaging in Pediatric Problems

Congenital anomalies. Young patients suspected of having malpositioned viscera or normal variations can be readily evaluated with liver

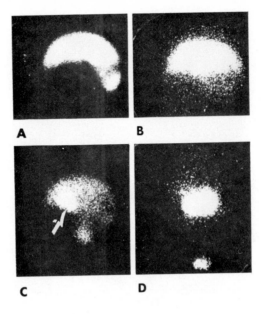

Fig. 7-3. (A) anterior colloid liver scintiphoto showing "symmetrical" liver and what appears to be low-lying spleen. (B) Early rose bengal excretion. (C) 1-hr ^{131}I-RB excretion demonstrating normal position of gallbladder (arrow). See text. (D) 24-hr ^{131}I-RB excretion showing normal bowel excretion.

imaging techniques. Situs inversus, polysplenia, asplenia, and symmetrical liver (Ivemark syndrome) can be rapidly and safely identified by these studies. Excretion studies with ^{131}I-RB often add useful information about the position of the gallbladder (midline in Ivemark, etc.) (Fig. 7-3). They also may reveal the identity of suspect masses in the region of the gallbladder fossa as normal variations of gallbladder position.

Intrinsic liver disease. Children with a variety of disease entities, including primary and secondary malignancies, abscesses, cysts, arteriovenous malformations, storage diseases, hepatitis, and even cardiac failure may present with hepatomegaly. Likewise, patients with abdominal masses or known primary malignant disease are often suspected of having liver involvement. The radiocolloid liver scintigram is a rapid and safe method for determining the architectural integrity of the liver (Fig. 7-4). Unfortunately, lesions under 2 cm in diameter are seen with difficulty, even with the newer detectors. While no statistics exist for pediatric error rates, Quinn has reported a "conservative" 19% error rate (7% false positive and 12% false negative) in adults with metastatic liver disease (5). In addition to this small lesion detection difficulty, image resolution may be degraded by respiratory motion of the liver during the

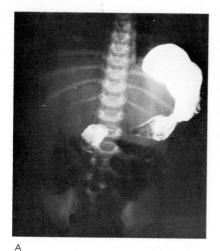

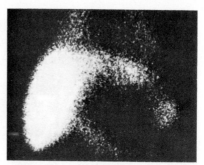

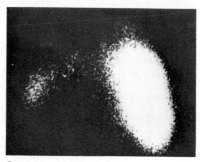

A

Fig. 7-4. (A) Upper GI x-ray showing abdominal mass displacing stomach laterally; Hepatomegaly? Left upper quadrant mass? (B) Colloid liver scintiphoto showing large defect from avascular mass in left lobe of liver. (Top is anterior view, bottom is posterior.) Surgery revealed intrahepatic neuroblastoma.

B

study. Lastly, normal variations of the liver contour may often be misleading (6). In spite of these limitations liver scintigraphy and the serum alkaline phosphatase remain the primary methods of screening patients with suspected primary or metastatic liver lesions (7–14), since other methods of liver evaluation have similar inaccuracy rates or more risk.

Liver imaging is clearly superior in the evaluation of patients with hepatic abscess (15–17). The study is sensitive, gives precise localization to the surgeon, and provides a useful means for treatment followup.

By combining the transmission lung scintigram with the emission (colloid) liver study, it is possible to localize subphrenic abscesses (18) (Fig. 7-5). Similarly, post-traumatic lacerations and collections can be quickly seen and followed (Fig. 7-6).

Patients with renal tumors can be evaluated by a combination of liver and renal scintigraphy as shown in Fig. 7-7. These studies are helpful in evaluating the nature and extent of the lesion.

A variety of benign conditions may be seen with liver scintigraphy, including the granulomatous disease associated with ulcerative colitis (Fig. 7-8). Likewise, patients with polycystic kidney disease frequently have cystic lesions in the liver (Fig. 7-9).

Following radiation therapy, a rather characteristic angular defect may be seen in the liver and should not be confused with actual tumor. Tumor may arise adjacent to or within the treatment area, as in the 20-

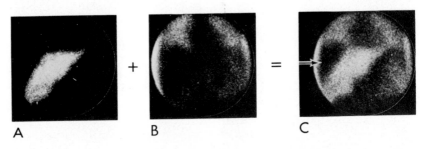

A   B   C

Fig. 7-5. (A) Colloid liver scintiphoto in 14-year-old girl with fever following appendectomy for ruptured appendix. (B) Transmission study in same patient showing cardiac silhouette, lungs, and lateral body walls. (C) A + B showing defect between liver and lungs and body wall, diagnostic of subphrenic mass. Subsequent drainage confirmed this as abscess. (Courtesy of James McRae, Donner Lab, Berkeley.)

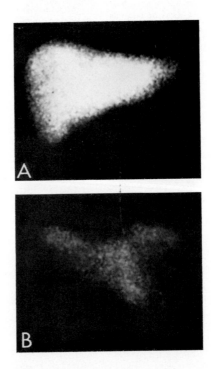

Fig. 7-6. Colloid liver scintiphotos in postsplenectomy patient who had been run over by automobile. (A) Anterior view (normal). (B) Posterior view showing posterolateral area of decreased activity in region of laceration seen at surgery.

year-old seen in Fig. 7-10. The discrepancy between the mass on plain radiograph of the abdomen and the liver scintiphoto led to the diagnosis of radiation-induced fibrosarcoma 19 years after radiation therapy for neuroblastoma. A similar case has been previously reported (19).

The jaundiced child. Initial enthusiasm for the use of radionuclides in differentiating patients suspected of having biliary atresia from neonatal hepatitis has progressed to confusion and disenchantment among pediatricians (20–25). The ^{131}I-RB study is useful, but experience has provided a better appreciation for the role of this procedure and how to prevent erroneous interpretation of the study (26–28).

We believe that a ^{99m}Tc-sulfur colloid liver scintiphoto study should always precede the ^{131}I-RB study. Recent attention has been called to

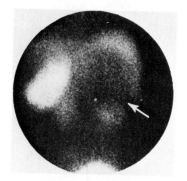

Fig. 7-7. Posterior liver/spleen scintiphoto combined with renal scintiphoto after injection of ^{99m}Tc-DTPA showing right suprarenal mass (arrow pointing to decreased activity) replacing superior pole of right kidney and extending well into posterior right lobe of liver. Surgically, ganglioneuroblastoma was found corresponding to defects on study. (Courtesy Shelby Miller, Los Angeles Children's Hospital.)

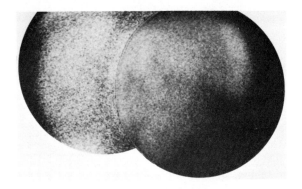

Fig. 7-8. Composite colloid liver scintiphoto showing hepatomegaly and diffuse irregularities in pattern of localization of material in young man with ulcerative colitis, confirmed pathologically as granulomatous disease of liver.

Anterior

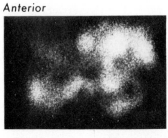

Posterior   *Right Lateral*

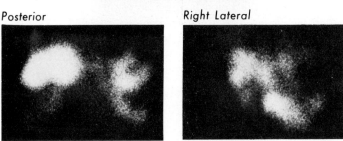

Fig. 7-9. Colloid liver scintiphotos in polycystic liver disease.

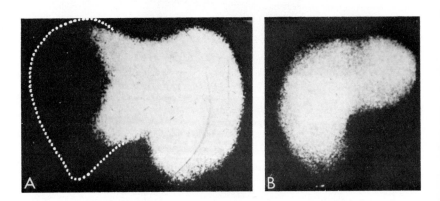

Fig. 7-10. 20-year-old man treated with 4,200 R for neuroblastoma at 1 year of age, presenting with abdominal pain and right upper quadrant mass on radiographic study. **(A)** Anterior colloid liver scintiphoto showing replacement of right lobe of liver by mass or fibrosis; **(B)** Right lateral view shows angular defect of right lobe mass anteriorly. (Pathology reported mass as compatible with radiation-induced fibrosarcoma.)

the value of this study in the diagnosis of obstructive jaundice. The pattern of dilated biliary radicles can frequently be discerned on the routine liver scan if special attention is given to the performance of the study (*29–30*). Heck and Gottschalk (*31*) advocate a breath-holding technique and have correctly identified 26 of 32 patients with dilated ducts in jaun-

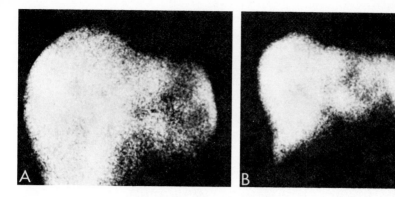

Fig. 7-11. Colloid liver scintiphoto. **(A)** Converging collimator. Anterior view demonstrating branching pattern of dilated intrahepatic bile ducts; **(B)** high-resolution collimator view of same patient.

diced patients with no false positives. "Gating" devices and computer techniques to improve resolution by minimizing breathing motion have been used with success (*32*). The pattern of dilated ducts is usually characteristic even without these special techniques (Fig. 7-11). It has been generally accepted that finding such a pattern on liver scan in a jaundiced patient is an indication for percutaneous cholangiography or surgery.

If the dilated duct pattern is seen on the colloid study and is followed by a pattern of absent bowel excretion on the ^{131}I-RB study, the probability of extrahepatic biliary obstruction (i.e., atresia or choledochal duct cyst) is high (Fig. 7-12). The presence of a large "cold" defect in the routine liver scintigram in the region of the porta hepatis is sufficient evidence to perform further studies to exclude the possibility of biliary obstruction.

Urinary excretion of ^{131}I-RB in patients with obstruction has previously been considered a potential "pitfall" (*33*). If, however, a background urine and daily 24-hr urine collections are made during the procedure, the total ^{131}I-RB urinary excretion can be evaluated. Increased urinary ^{131}I-RB may correlate with the degree of liver disease, as had been predicted by an early report (*34*). In addition, we scan over the renal area in patients suspected of having obstruction and in patients with high urinary excretion of the isotope to prevent confusion of the renal outline with the bowel excretion of ^{131}I-RB.

Patients who have markedly abnormal clearance curves [greater than 86% retention in the Nordyke series (*4*)] have been considered to have liver failure whether or not they have excretion into the gut. These patients may show prompt excretion to the GI tract or delayed passage and therefore should be followed at 48, 72 hr, or longer. Their urine will

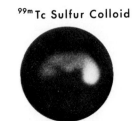

99mTc Sulfur Colloid

Anterior

131I Rose Bengal

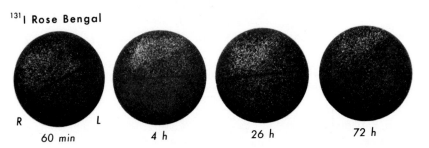

R   L

60 min   4 h   26 h   72 h

Fig. 7-12. Colloid liver scintiphoto demonstrating "cold" defect in porta and linear branching of dilated ducts toward porta with splenomegaly in patient with extrahepatic biliary atresia. ^{131}I-RB study shows no excretion. (Courtesy of Robert Hattner, UCSF.)

show an increased excretion of the ^{131}I-RB but *generally* less activity than those patients with mechanical obstruction (see Table 7-1).

Patients with complete obstructive biliary tract disease may show any degree of abnormal blood clearance of ^{131}I-RB but will demonstrate no evidence of excretion into the bowel at intervals of 72 hr or more. They will have the highest values of urinary excretion. These findings have been the subject of many reports, particularly in pediatric patients (*35–39*). Decreased stool excretion mirrors the absent bowel activity, and therefore stool counting is rarely performed. (It is quite difficult to obtain an uncontaminated stool sample in the neonate.) Occasional patients with severe hepatocellular disease may simulate obstruction on both scintigrams and urinary excretion. In our experience, patients with drug-induced toxic hepatitis (e.g., from immuran or chlorpromazine) as well as severe neonatal hepatitis have shown identical urinary excretion and scintiphoto study results as patients with partial or complete mechanical obstruction (*40*).

Patients with good bowel excretion of ^{131}I-RB and 60–86% retention of the radionuclide on a clearance study fall into a large class of patients of "indeterminate etiology" including acute hepatitis and varying degrees of obstruction. Their urinary excretion of ^{131}I-RB should be normal.

While some authors have used more elaborate techniques (*41–42*), we have felt that the simplified, uniform procedure encompassing the parameters discussed is preferable. A pre-injection drink of Lugol's solution is given routinely to block thyroidal uptake of ^{131}I, and a fasting state is maintained to facilitate gallbladder visualization.

Specialized use of the ^{131}I-RB study has been suggested by case reports, including one patient with a "functional" hepatoma that concentrated ^{131}I-RB (*43*) and a patient in whom bile leakage was studied with ^{131}I-RB (*44*).

Using similar rose bengal techniques, a recent report indicates four patients misdiagnosed in a series of 25 (*28*). To categorize patients with liver disease into "surgical" and "medical" jaundice, all the parameters discussed above may be necessary.

It is apparent that the ^{131}I-RB study must be performed and evaluated with care and correlated with other studies, including colloid liver scintigraphy. In our hands, the normal study and the pattern of dilated ducts of extrahepatic biliary obstruction remain the only "certainties".

Newer, more specific agents for visualizing the biliary tract are in the developmental stage but their clinical value will need further evaluation.

The ^{131}I-RB examination has been criticized, particularly in the pediatric age group, because of the radiation exposure. Sharp, using the Brookhaven nomogram (based on a dose of 1 μCi of ^{131}I-RB/kg), states that the normal liver will receive 2.1 mrads and the patient with biliary atresia 19.8 mrad (*35*). These values are not in excess of those routinely accepted in other diagnostic procedures, such as GI tract radiography, intravenous pyelography, and cardiac catheterization. We have used a dose in the range of 25–50 μCi of ^{131}I-RB with children. As mentioned, we suggest routine thyroidal blockage by a preinjection drink of Lugol's solution. Repeated doses of Lugol's on succeeding days for blocking may be necessary if biliary obstruction is found.

Summary

Liver imaging techniques with presently available equipment can provide the pediatrician with valuable information about the size, shape, and integrity of the liver, and assist in assessing extent of abdominal masses. A variety of diseases have characteristic patterns, and these should be appreciated, particularly that of branching, dilated intrahepatic radicals. Cautious use of the ^{131}I-RB study can assist in further evaluation, particularly in the jaundiced child. Correlation with the clinical problem is essential to maximize the effectiveness of these studies.

References

1. ADELSTEIN, SJ: The risk:benefit ratio in nuclear medicine. *Hosp Practice* 8: 141–149, 1973

2. SORENSON LB, ARCHAMBAULT M: Visualization of the liver by scanning with Mo⁹⁹ (molybdate) as tracer. *J Lab Clin Med* 62: 330–340, 1963

3. LOWENSTEIN JL: Radioactive rose bengal test as a quantitative measure of liver function. *Proc Soc Exp Biol Med* 93: 377–378, 1956

4. NORDYKE RA, BLAHD WH: Blood disappearance of radioactive rose bengal—rapid simple test of liver function. *JAMA* 170: 1159–1164, 1959

5. QUINN JL: Use of diagnostic nuclear medicine procedures in breast cancer. *Cancer* 28: 1695–1698, 1971

6. KATZ, HJ, WILLIAM AJ: Accessory lobes of the liver and their significance in roentgen diagnosis. *Ann Intern Med* 116: 95–110, 1965

7. MCAFEE JG, AUSE RG, WAGNER HN: Diagnostic value of scintillation scanning of the liver. *Arch Intern Med* 116: 95–110, 1965

8. GOTTSCHALK A: Liver scanning. *JAMA* 200: 630–633, 1967

9. SIBER FJ: Scintillation scanning as an aid in the diagnosis of liver disease. *Lahey Clinic Foundation Bull* 17: 7–12, 1968

10. SMITH LB, WILLIAMS RD: The relative diagnostic accuracy of liver radioactive isotope photoscanning. *Arch Surg* 96: 693–697, 1968

11. FERRIER FL, HATCHER CR, ACHORD JL, et al: The value of liver scanning for detection of metastatic cancer. *Am Surg* 35: 112–120, 1969

12. WILSON FE, PRESTON DF, OVERHOLT EL: Detection of hepatic neoplasm: Hepatic scanning combined with liver-function studies. *JAMA* 209: 676–679, 1969

13. COVINGTON EE: The accuracy of liver photoscans. *Am J Roentgenol Radium Ther Nucl Med* 109: 742–744, 1970

14. JHINGRAN SG, JORDAN L, JAHNS MF, et al: Liver scintigrams compared with alkaline phosphatase and BSP determinations in the detection of metastatic carcinoma. *J Nucl Med* 12: 227–230, 1971

15. CUARON A, GORDON F: Liver scanning: Analysis of 2500 cases of amebic hepatic abscesses. *J Nucl Med* 11: 435–439, 1970

16. IIO M, IUCHI M, KITANI K, et al: Scintigraphic evaluation of the liver with Schistosomiasis japonica. *J Nucl Med* 12: 655–659, 1971

17. LAZARCHICK J, DESOUZA E, DESILVA NA, et al: Pyogenic liver abscess. *Mayo Clin Proc* 48: 349–355, 1973

18. VOLPE JA, MCRAE J, JOHNSTON GS: Transmission scintigraphy in the evaluation of subphrenic abscess. *Am J Roentgenol Radium Ther Nucl Med* 109: 733–734, 1970

19. Case Records of the Massachusetts General Hospital, Case 17, 1972 *N Engl J Med* 286: 934–940, 1972

20. NORDYKE RA, BLAHD WH: The differential diagnosis of biliary tract obstruction with radioactive rose bengal. *J Lab Clin Med* 51: 565–579, 1958

21. NORDYKE RA: Biliary tract obstruction and its localization with radio-iodinated rose bengal. *Am J Gastroenterol* 33: 563–573, 1960

22. BRENT RL, GEPPERT LJ: The use of radioactive rose bengal in the evaluation of infantile jaundice. *Am J Dis Child* 98: 720–730, 1959

23. GHADIMI H, SASS-KORTSAK A: Evaluation of the radioactive rose bengal test for the differential diagnosis of obstruction jaundice in infants. *N Engl J Med* 265: 351–358, 1961

24. KAWAGUCHI M, SOBLE AR, BERK JE: Studies with I¹³¹-labeled rose bengal. I. Derivation of a technic for use in the differential diagnosis of jaundice. *Am J Dig Dis* 7: 289–299, 1962

25. KAWAGUCHI M, BERK JE, SOBLE AR: Studies with I¹³¹-labeled rose bengal. II. Clinical evaluation of a modified technic for differential diagnosis of jaundice. *Am J Dig Dis* 7: 300–308, 1962

26. NORDYKE RA: Radioiodinated rose bengal in liver and biliary tract function testing: a reappraisal. *Gastroenterology* 39: 258–260, 1960

27. SCHUMAN BM, REYNOLDS WA, EYLER WR: The limitations of the I¹³¹ rose bengal liver function test in the differential diagnosis of jaundice. *Gastroenterology* 45: 73–76, 1963

28. SILVERBERG M, ROSENTHALL L, FREEMAN LM: Rose Bengal excretion studies as an aid in the differential diagnosis of neonatal jaundice. *Semin Nucl Med* 3: 69–80, 1973

29. ARTER W, MORRIS JG, MCRAE J, et al: Liver scanning in obstructive jaundice using colloidal radiogold. *J Coll Radiol Austr* 9: 68–77, 1965

30. GAMMILL SL, MAXFIELD WS, FONT RG, et al: Filling defects on scintillation scans of the liver associated with dilatation of the bile ducts. *Am J Roentgenol Radium Ther Nucl Med* 108: 37–42, 1969

31. HECK LL, GOTTSCHALK A: The appearance of intrahepatic biliary duct dilatation on the liver scan. *Radiology* 99: 135–140, 1971

32. OPPENHEIM BE: A method using a digital computer for reducing respiratory artifact on liver scans made with a camera. *J Nucl Med* 12: 625–628, 1971

33. FREEMAN LM, KAY CJ, DERMAN A: Renal excretion of radioiodinated rose bengal—a pitfall in the interpretation of rose bengal abdominal scans. *J Nucl Med* 9: 227–232, 1968

34. BRENT RL, GEPPERT LJ: The use of radioactive rose bengal in the evaluation of infantile jaundice. *Am J Dis Child* 98: 720–730, 1959

35. SHARP HL, KRIVIT W, LOWMAN, JT: The diagnosis of complete extrahepatic obstruction by rose bengal I¹³¹. *J Pediatr* 70: 46–53, 1967

36. NORDYKE RA: Surgical vs nonsurgical jaundice: Differentiation by a combination of rose bengal I¹³¹ and standard liver-function tests. *JAMA* 194: 949–953, 1965

37. EYLER WR, DUSAULT LA, POZNANSKI AK, et al: Isotope scanning in the evaluation of jaundiced patients. *Radiol Clin North Am* 4: 589–603, 1966

38. EYLER WR, DUSAULT LA, POZNANSKI AK, et al: Liver scanning with special reference to jaundiced patients. *Lahey Clinic Bull* 17: 13–20, 1968

39. BURKE G, HALKO A: Dynamic clinical studies with radioisotopes and the scintillation camera. II. Rose Bengal I¹³¹ liver function studies. *JAMA* 198: 608–618, 1966

40. HANDMAKER H: Unpublished data, 1971

41. WHITING EG, NUSYNOWITZ ML: Radioactive rose bengal testing in the differential diagnosis of jaundice. *Surg Gynecol Obstet* 127: 729–733, 1968

42. MENA I, KIVEL R, MAHONEY P, et al: A method for increasing the sensitivity of the rose bengal I¹³¹ liver function test with the use of bromsulphalein. *J Lab Clin Med* 54: 167–173, 1959

43. SHOOP JD: Functional hepatoma demonstrated with rose bengal scanning. *Am J Roentgenol Radium Ther Nucl Med* 107: 51–53, 1969

44. SPENCER RP, KAPLAN MM, GLENN WL: Use of I¹³¹-rose bengal to follow bile leakage: report of a case. *Am J Dig Dis* 12: 1169–1173, 1967

Chapter 8

Spleen

Gerald S. Freedman

Careful examination of the left upper quadrant of the pediatric patient will usually disclose the presence or absence of an enlarged spleen. Although the spleen has a wide variation in weight and mobility, the normal spleen rarely extends below the left costal margin. While the presence of a palpable spleen is usually of pathological significance, the wide variation in splenic weight and position may make the detection of splenomegaly difficult on routine physical examination. When present, it may be difficult to differentiate the enlarged spleen from other palpable masses in the left upper quadrant. For these reasons, radionuclide imaging of the spleen has become a simple and valuable method for precisely locating and establishing the accurate size of functioning splenic tissue. The size and weight of the spleen can be approximated by direct measurement from the scan; normal values have been established based on the splenic length and the age and weight of the child (1, 2) (Table 8-1).

TABLE 8-1.   Relationship of Pediatric Spleen Length to Weight and Age

Length (cm) = 5.7 + 0.31 A* (Ref. 1)
Weight (gm) = 24 + 7 A (Ref. 2)
Weight (gm) = 22.6 L − 104 (Ref. 1)
Length (cm) = 2.3 + 0.05 H* (Ref. 1)

* A = age in years; H = height in centimeters.

Normal Splenic Function

In fetal life the spleen serves as one of the primary sites for production of formed elements of blood. Soon after birth this role is taken over by the normal bone marrow. The spleen thereafter is capable of performing several functions in its spongelike mass of sinusoids, reticulum framework, and lymphoid tissue.

1. The primary splenic function appears to be the destruction and extraction from the circulation of aged, damaged, or otherwise altered formed elements of the blood. When this physiological role is exaggerated, anemia, leukopenia, and thrombocytopenia can occur. This is called "hypersplenism".
2. Another fundamental role of the spleen is as part of the body defense system of lymphoid tissue. It produces lymphocytes and immature plasma cells which are involved with cellular and humoral immunity.
3. Finally, the spleen retains its potential as a site for extramedullary hematopoiesis. Under appropriate stress, the sinusoids of the red pulp exhibit increased cellularity and produce normoblasts, megakaryocytes, and myeloid cells.

Although well supported by its two ligaments (the gastrosplenic and lienorenal) and resting on a third (costocolic), the spleen is often quite mobile. Displacement due to gastric dilatation has been reported (3) and its intra-abdominal movement has been described as the "wandering spleen" (4). The spleen's position on its pedicle is variable, and the position of the hilum is also variable. A case has been described exhibiting "the upside-down spleen" (5).

Choice of Radiopharmaceuticals

The spleen's ability to sequester and extract damaged red blood cells in the sinuses and to phagocytize colloidal material in the reticuloendothelial cells provides two physiological mechanisms for splenic evaluation. Table 8-2 lists several agents which can be used to exploit these physiological properties of the spleen. In most institutions, the standard method is to label the red blood cells with ^{51}Cr (sodium chromate) and then damage the erythrocytes with heat treatment. This is an acceptable method, but results may be quite unpredictable with variable hepatic and splenic sequestration. Moreover, since only 9% of the ^{51}Cr emissions are detectable gammas, even a relatively small administered dose results in considerable radiation to the spleen. The stannous chloride method of labeling red blood cells with ^{99m}Tc has recently been described (6). Ex-

TABLE 8-2. Spleen Imaging Agents

Radiopharmaceutical	Administered dose (μCi/kg)
RBC labels	
^{51}Cr	5
^{99m}Tc	30
Colloids	
^{99m}Tc-S-colloid	50
^{113m}In	50
^{198}Au	2.5

cess stannous chloride appears to simultaneously damage the red blood cells in a predictable way and assists in the binding of the technetium. The preliminary clinical report is encouraging and future experience is awaited with interest. These labels permit isolation and visualization of splenic tissue and are valuable when the spleen is obscured by overlying liver tissue or when ectopic or splenic regrowth is to be evaluated. However, the need to label the patient's own red blood cells makes these procedures somewhat more complicated.

A simpler, although less specific, method of visualizing the spleen is the use of a radioactive colloid. Historically, ^{198}Au was used with a small colloidal size (about 1 mμ). This small size resulted in a higher concentration in hepatic tissue than in splenic tissue. The introduction of technetium-labeled-sulfur colloid (particles about 1 micron) provides a more even liver-spleen distribution of colloid in the two organs. When using this material, more than 90% of the colloid is extracted from the blood by the RE cells within 15 min and imaging can proceed. The radiation dose to the patient per millicurie injected is a function of age and is given in Table 8-3.

Patient Positioning

When possible, an anterior, posterior, and left lateral view of the spleen should be performed. In addition to these routine views, a left anterior-oblique view is often helpful since the left lobe of the liver is frequently superimposed over the splenic area. Counts over each organ to determine the liver/spleen ratio are also recommended. With younger, uncooperative children a study with the rectilinear scanner may prolong the examination, and for this reason the gamma camera is preferred. It permits more views in a shorter time period. The anxious and combative child can be held against the reassuring bosom of the parent while the camera views are being obtained. Figure 8-1 shows the conventional views of the normal spleen.

TABLE 8-3. I.V. ^{99m}Tc-Sulfur Colloid Absorbed Dose (mrads/mCi)*

Organ	Age (yr)					
	Birth	1	5	10	15	Adult
Total body	180	65	43	29	19	15
Liver	2,100–2,700	1,030–1,320	630–815	435–560	330–420	240–310
Spleen	4,950–1,650	1,590–530	960–320	600–200	450–150	370–123
Male gonads	200	70	45	30	20	17
Female gonads	250	80	50	35	25	21
Red marrow						72–36

* Semin Nucl Med 3: 55–68, 1973

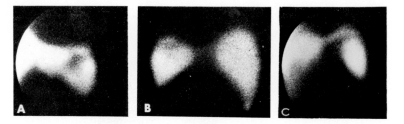

Fig. 8-1. (A) Anterior and (B) posterior views of spleen show area of decreased activity. (C) Left anterior oblique view shows this is due to extension of left lobe of liver over spleen rather than splenic defect.

Clinical Applications

Left upper quadrant mass. In the evaluation of a left upper quadrant mass one must consider the following possible causes:

1. splenomegaly
2. pancreatic mass
3. renal mass
4. gastric mass
5. colonic mass
6. retroperitoneal tumor or
7. superficial neoplasm.

The spleen scan is a simple, direct approach to this differential diagnosis. In addition to documenting frank splenic enlargement and displacement, the presence of a mass within the spleen can also be seen. Moreover, the relative distribution of activity between the liver and the spleen can be a useful measure of hypersplenism. Often the liver, kidney, or retroperitoneal mass will displace the spleen, and an analysis of the splenic position can often indicate the nature of the displacing mass. While the spleen may be considered a retroperitoneal organ, it behaves

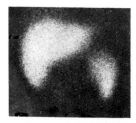 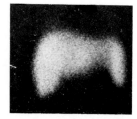

Fig. 8-2. Splenic mobility. (Left) Study done when child had gastric distention. (Right) Study done 2 days later after gastric decompression shows spleen was displaced downward in earlier study. (Reprinted with permission from Ref. *3*)

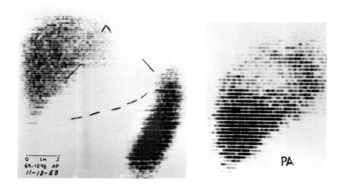

Fig. 8-3 (Left). Splenic displacement due to retroperitoneal sarcoma.

Fig. 8-4 (Right). Defect presumed to be Hodgkin's involvement of the spleen. (Reprinted with permission from Ref. *11.*)

more like an intraperitoneal organ, thrust into the peritoneal cavity, somewhat moveable on its pedicle. Splenic mobility secondary to a dilated stomach (Fig. 8-2) and a retroperitoneal sarcoma (Fig. 8-3) can be demonstrated. Table 8-4 is a list of causes of splenomegaly. They are divided into minimal, moderate, and massive.

Lymphoma, leukemia, and other malignancies. These diseases may be considered as myeloproliferative disorders. Massive splenomegaly is often seen in the chronic forms. The detection and staging of some of these may be aided by spleen scanning. Unfortunately, preoperative spleen scanning has proven to be relatively insensitive in the documentation of Hodgkin's involvement of the spleen. Surgical pathology specimens often show small or microscopic Hodgkin's involvement undetectable by splenic scanning. In many cases confirmation of splenomegaly and the exact location of the spleen was of considerable help to the therapist. In these patients an anterior and posterior spleen scan is preferred so that the cutaneous landmarks can be drawn for the therapist. The rare secondary involvement of the spleen by metastatic tumors is

---

TABLE 8-4. Causes of Splenomegaly

Minimal	Moderate	Massive
1. Hepatitis	1. Cirrhosis	1. Thalassemia
2. Bacterial endocarditis	2. Hodgkin's disease	2. Malaria
3. Pyelonephritis	3. Leukemia	3. Leukemia
4. Pneumonia	4. Hematoma	4. Myeloid metaplasia
5. Mononucleosis	5. Portal vein thrombosis	5. Cyst
6. Cystic fibrosis	6. Infarction	6. Glycogen storage disease

remarkable (Fig. 8-4). Considering the propensity for scavenging cellular material, this observation may be significant. Do the phagocytic cells of the spleen neutralize or ingest the neoplastic cells? Does the immunological capacity of the spleen neutralize these neoplastic cells?

A review of the tumor registry in The Memorial Hospital and Andersen series of 768 benign and 175 malignancies in children failed to reveal a single metastasis or primary splenic neoplasm (excluding lymphomas). In adults angiosarcomas and lymphosarcomas have been reported in the spleen. In a mixed series of 6,851 autopsies on adult patients with cancer only 1.8% (125 cases) had splenic involvement (7).

Anemia and blood dyscrasias. Exaggerated destruction of blood elements can produce a pancytopenia or a selective anemia, leukopenia, or thrombocytopenia. It may be a primary process, or secondary to infection or other cause. Excessive production of RBCs, as in polycythemia, is also possible. In some conditions such as spherocytosis, sickle cell disease, thalassemia, and combinations of sickle cell and thalassemia, these altered red blood cells fall prey to the natural phagocytic activity of the spleen. In other conditions such as idiopathic thrombocytopenic purpura, for unknown reasons, hypersplenism can dangerously reduce the platelet level. Splenectomy is often curative in these cases of hypersplenism. Postsplenectomy platelet, white blood cell, and red blood cell levels can

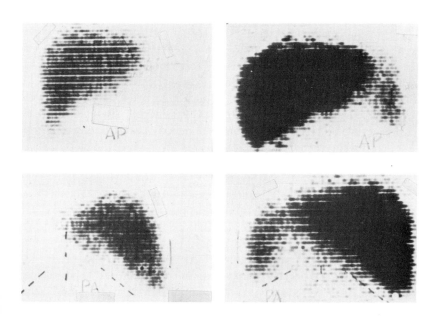

Fig. 8-5. Sickle cell disease. (Left) Anterior (upper) and posterior (lower) views show absent splenic function. (Right) Five days later following extensive transfusions spleen is visualized. (Reprinted with permission from Ref. *8.*)

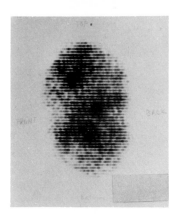

Fig. 8-6. Surgical specimen spleen scan shows
multiple infarcted areas in Cooley's anemia.
(Reprinted with permission from Ref. *11*.)

often return to normal. Accessory splenic tissue, in common with the
main organ, is derived from the main mesogastrium. One or more accessory spleens is present in 25% of children (*4*). Occasionally there
may be a recurrence of a significant anemia following splenectomy due
to hypertrophy of residual splenic tissue. In these cases, a spleen scan
is extremely valuable in determining if accessory splenic tissue is present.
For this purpose, labeled red blood cells are favored over colloids because there is no interference from overlying hepatic activity.

In some conditions excessive sequestration of red blood cells of the
spleen can completely "clog" the splenic pulp and produce a "functional
asplenia". Pearson and colleagues (*8*) recently have shown the reversibility of functional asplenia in children with sickle cell anemia. Figure
8-5 demonstrates the appearance of functioning splenic tissue in a child
with sickle cell disease. The spleen was "de-sludged" by repeated transfusions of whole blood. This return of function is short-lived and is usually lost within several months.

In Cooley's anemia (thalassemia) significant splenomegaly will occur when the hemoglobin drops below 8 gm/100 ml (Fig. 8-6). If splenectomy is performed, the patients are susceptible to overwhelming infections due to pneumococcus, meningococcus, or H. influenzae. The
indications for splenectomy are: (A) increasing need for transfusion, (B)
massive splenomegaly, and (C) decreased donor RBC survival (less than
18 days).

Infection and portal hypertension. Splenomegaly and hypersplenism
can result from a wide variety of bacterial and viral infections. While
malaria and parasitic infections account for most of the splenomegaly on
a global basis, they are rarely seen in the United States although they
must always be considered (Fig. 8-7). Pathologically, splenomegaly associated with systemic infection results in an increased number of white

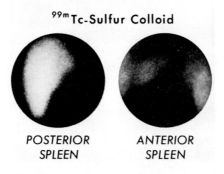

POSTERIOR
SPLEEN

ANTERIOR
SPLEEN

Fig. 8-7. Splenomegaly in returning Peace Corps volunteer
with malaria. (Courtesy of H. Handmaker.)

blood cells and reticuloendothelial cells which engorge the red pulp. If
secondary hypersplenism occurs with leukopenia and thrombocytopenia
and if biopsy of the marrow is normal, then splenectomy should be considered. Occasionally, hepatitis can produce splenomegaly during the
infectious phase and later produce a postnecrotic cirrhosis resulting in
portal hypertension. Secondarily, the increased portal pressure is transmitted back to the splenic venous system and produces congestive
splenomegaly and neutropenia (Banti's syndrome). Histologically,
splenic sinuses are dilated with increased fibrous tissue within red pulp.
Some common causes of cirrhosis and portal hypertension are: (A) Wilson's disease, (B) rheumatic heart disease, (C) biliary atresia, (D) Budd-
Chiari syndrome, and (E) cystic fibrosis. Figure 8-8 is an example of
splenomegaly secondary to the cirrhosis of chronic congestive heart failure. Occasionally the phagocytic property of the spleen comes up against

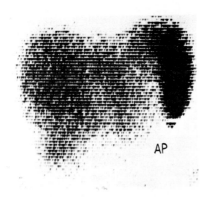

AP

Fig. 8-8. Hepatosplenomegaly with shift of colloid to spleen due to
portal hypertension secondary to CHF from rheumatic heart disease.

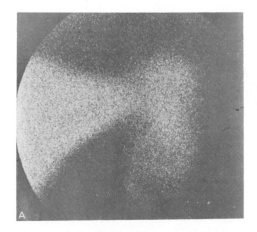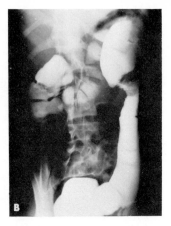

Fig. 8-9. (A) Spleen scintiphoto shows defect at inferior margin. (B) Barium enema shows narrowing at splenic flexure due to inflammatory response to splenic abscess.

a nondigestible infection. In these cases the spleen can become the site of a splenic abscess. Spleen scan shows characteristic splenomegaly with one or more filling defects. Figure 8-9 shows multiple splenic abscesses secondary to E. coli and secondary inflammatory narrowing of the colonic splenic flexure, which required segmental excision at laparotomy.

Trauma, surgery, and irradiation. Although somewhat protected by the left lower thoracic rib cage, the spleen is sensitive to blunt trauma. This can often produce intracapsular hemorrhage, thrombosis, or a fatal laceration. When splenic trauma is suspected, all standard and special angle views of the spleen should be used. One or more should include a surface skin marker. Occasionally a traumatic bleed will not result in a visible intrasplenic defect but can be diagnosed only by the displacement of the spleen from the rib margin caused by the enlarging hematoma. Figure 8-10 shows an intrasplenic filling defect caused by traumatic

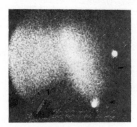

Fig. 8-10. Irregular lateral splenic margin and increasing distance from flank marker (white dots) due to traumatic subcapsular hematoma.

hematoma. Prompt laparotomy and splenectomy is the only reliable cure for a traumatized spleen. When the fear of hemorrhage due to unfavorable clotting characteristics is a contraindication for needed splenectomy, splenic artery ligation may be considered. Resulting involution of the ischemic splenic tissue often gives good results, and the splenic reduction can be documented by spleen scan. The viability of the residual splenic tissue is usually maintained by collaterals from the left gastric and the superior mesenteric arteries. Another interesting surgical application is the transposition of the spleen into the left thorax as an attempt to provide collateral venous pathways in Budd-Chiari syndrome, as reported by Strauch (9). This case resulted in a functional asplenia by spleen scan.

Finally, the relative radiosensitivity of the reticuloendothelial cells can be monitored by serial spleen scan following irradiation of the spleen for a variety of myeloproliferative disorders (11).

Primary reticuloendothelial granuloma and cysts. These diseases often produce massive splenomegaly. Under the reticuloses are included: (A) Gaucher's (Fig. 8-11) and (B) Niemann-Pick which are lipid storage diseases seen in children, (C) Letterer-Siwe, (D) Schuller-Christian, and (E) eosinophilic granuloma which are non-lipid storage diseases. While primary cysts of the spleen are uncommon they usually present as a large filling defect in a massive spleen (Fig. 8-12).

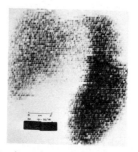

Fig. 8-11. Massive splenomegaly due to Gaucher's disease.

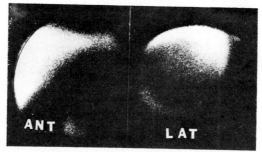

Fig. 8-12. Splenic cyst. Note inferior band of normal splenic tissue.

References

1. Spencer R, Pearson R, Lange R: Human spleen: scan studies on growth and response to medication. *J Nucl Med* 12: 466–468, 1971

2. Seltzer RA, Kereiakes JG, Saenger EL: Radiation exposure from radio-isotopes in pediatrics. *N Engl J Med* 271: 84–90, 1964

3. Landgarten S, Spencer R: Splenic displacement due to gastric dilation. *J Nucl Med* 13: 223–224, 1972

4. Bailey H, Love M: *Short Practice of Surgery,* London, H K Lewis & Co, Ltd, 1959, pp 370–391

5. Westcott JL, Krufky EL: Upside down spleen. *Radiology* 105: 517–521, 1972

6. Eckleman W, Richards P, Atkins HL, et al: Visualization of the human spleen with ⁹⁹ᵐTc-labeled red blood cells. *J Nucl Med* 12: 310–311, 1971

7. Dargeon HW, *Tumors of Children.* New York, PB Hoeber, 1960, p 223

8. Pearson H, Cornelius E, Schwartz A, et al: Transfusion-reversible functional asplenia in young children with sickle cell anemia. *N Engl J Med* 283: 334–337, 1970

9. Strauch G: Supradiaphragmatic splenic transposition. *Am J Surg* 119: 379–384, 1970

10. Spencer R: Personal communication, 1973

11. Freedman G, Spencer R, Weinraub G: *Radionuclide Evaluation of Splenic Disease and Function.* Chicago, Ill, Micro X-ray Recorder Film Slide Division (slide course).

Discussion

Peter E. Valk (Donner Laboratory, Berkeley, Calif.): You mentioned in passing the use of ⁹⁹ᵐTc-RBC for spleen imaging. In 1970–71, McRae and I studied over 70 patients at Sydney University by such a method, using the stannous ion to label the cells and heat to damage them, and obtaining rapid and high splenic uptake without interfering activity in the liver or blood pool. Although most splenic abnormalities can be detected with colloids, we found a number of cases where the abnormality could only be shown by the red cell method. In particular, in one patient with hemolytic anemia who had responded to splenectomy and subsequently relapsed, we were able to show an accessory spleen which was not imaged with colloid.

Dr. Freedman: Thank you for sharing your experience with us. The recent papers describing the Tc-stannous method of labeling RBCs are encouraging but only cover a few cases. Splenic labeling specificity using excess stannous ion will have to be compared to heat damage to determine the best method.

Daniel Schere (Children's Hospital, Buenos Aires, Argentina): Do you have any experience in micropolysplenia? It is another indication for spleen scans. We have studied a couple of newborns with congenital heart disease. There were no Howell-Jolly bodies and we were not able to demonstrate their spleens with ^{51}Cr-RBC.

Dr. Freedman: I have not seen a case of micropolysplenia demonstrated with a radionuclide study. With the expected widespread use of ^{99m}Tc-labeled RBCs to specifically label splenic tissue we will have a better chance to study this entity.

John D. Keyes, Jr. (Mercy Hospital, Redding, Calif.): Re: Paucity of metastases in spleen. Metastases to spleen are very uncommon which is why there are few reported cases. Lymphomatous lesions are doubtless the result of multicentric involvement.

Dr. Freedman: The Children's Tumor Registry in Memorial Hospital and Andersen's series of 768 "benign" and 175 malignant neoplasms (excluding lymphoma) showed no involvement of the spleen (Dargeon HW, *Tumors of Children.* New York, PB Hoeber, 1960, p 223). This observation is certainly striking and one can only speculate as to the reason for this neoplastic protection. Obviously something is going on which we as yet do not understand.

J. D. Shoop (University of New Mexico, Albuquerque, N.M.): Have you seen hepatization of spleen in biliary atresia? We have seen such a case.

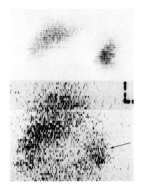

(Upper) ^{99m}Tc-sulfur colloid anterior scintigram of liver and spleen in 5-month-old child with surgically proven complete biliary atresia and cirrhosis, and enlarged spleen. (Lower) ^{131}I-rose bengal anterior scan showing splenic uptake of material corresponding to colloid uptake (arrow).

Dr. Freedman: We have not seen splenic uptake of ^{131}I-rose bengal in about a dozen patients we have studied with biliary atresia. Since the ^{131}I-rose bengal is seen in the mid abdomen, the possibility of a collection in the small bowel must always be considered in these cases. Moreover, the kidney is an alternate pathway of excretion for rose bengal. Caution must be exercised when calling left upper quadrant activity "hepatization of the spleen".

R. Hattner (University of California, San Francisco, Calif.): Do you, by the use of the term "hypersplenism", imply the condition commonly accepted to be constituted by peripherally decreased formed elements, or shortened fractional disappearance time thereof? If not, what do you mean?

Dr. Freedman: By hypersplenism we mean exaggeration of the spleen's phagocytic or sequestration ability. It is usually manifest by some form of anemia or cytopenia. The liver/spleen ratio can be used as an index of the distribution of colloid and as such is a measure of hypersplenism.

S. W. Miller (Children's Hospital, Los Angeles, Calif.): Infarcts or subcapsular hematomas may be well visualized on a flow study.

Dr. Freedman: I agree, thank you.

Dr. Chin (Emory University, Atlanta, Ga.): Abdominal anatomic features can be marked in a camera photo with lead strip or [57]Co-labeled tubing.

Dr. Freedman: Our preference for the scanner in the cooperative patient is because it allows the physician not only to mark the costal margin and anatomical features but also more likely results in the physician rather than the technician marking the patient.

Dr. Chin: We have confirmed functional spleens with C. Dinward, including impaired uptake of heat-damaged ^{51}Cr-labeled cells.

Dr. Freedman: I believe this has also been done at Yale by H. Pearson.

Dr. Hattner: You have offered increased splenic transit time as an explanation for relatively increased splenic activity in colloid scintigraphy. Would you not be inclined to agree that equally likely, or at least certainly not dismissable, would be that decreased hepatic perfusion, resulting in prolonged plasma disappearance given unchanged splenic extraction efficiency, and therefore larger integral dose, resulting in relatively increased activity, represents an additional consideration?

Dr. Freedman: Activity present in any organ is a function of the amount brought there by the blood and the amount extracted by the organ from the blood. With liver damage and increased portal pressure, less activity may be cleared by the liver leaving higher blood levels to be available for other RE tissue. Portal hypertension will result in increased pressure in the splenic vein and splenic pulp which will probably cause a slower passage of the colloid through the spleen. Both of these hypotheses contribute to the relative increase in activity in the spleen compared with the liver.

Chapter **9**

Kidney

James J. Conway and R. Bruce Filmer

The clinical applications of radionuclide techniques to pediatric urology have been described in a number of papers (*1–9*). Some of the earlier reports on the use of renography, renal imaging, and cystography in children were derived from a limited experience. It is difficult, if not impossible, to evaluate the efficacy of a new technique based upon such limited experience, particularly when one considers the many variables involved in clinical situations. One must also be cautious of accepting a new diagnostic technique since the actual clinical value may be obscured by the enthusiasm of the innovator. As a result, the initial enthusiasm for a technique may wane when a significant clinical value fails to materialize in day-to-day practice.

We felt that a review of our extensive clinical experience might provide some definitive indications for the practical use of these techniques. Thus it is the purpose of this chapter to present a review and to indicate the usefulness of radionuclide renography, renal imaging, and cystography in the daily clinical practice of pediatric urology.

Material

A review of approximately 600 renal studies and 250 bladder studies was correlated with the clinical followup derived from the patient's chart. The review was conducted with the assistance of a pediatric urologist (RBF) whose knowledge of his speciality and of the patient's clinical problem provided an insight greater than that provided by the chart alone. In each instance the considerations were: (A) Did the test alter the patient's diagnosis, therapy, or the eventual outcome from that expected? and (B) was the test necessary? The answers, of course, were subjective in many instances and at best, only an overall impression was achieved. Factors of importance will be illustrated and discussed here.

Methods

In nuclear medicine, probably more so than in any other diagnostic field, there has been an almost constant evolution of technique brought about by the continuing introduction of newer radiopharmaceuticals, imaging devices, and methods of analysis. The techniques used in this study are described in this section.

The renogram. Our procedure bears little resemblance to the original renogram technique introduced by Taplin (*10*) and Winter (*11*) in 1956. Early renogram methods were fraught with difficulty due to misplacement of probes, field overlap, probe imbalance, ectopic location of renal tissue, and numerous other factors. In addition, there was a tendency to ascribe detailed functional significance to the various portions of the renogram curve, i.e., vascular, secretory, and excretory phases. Each phase, how-

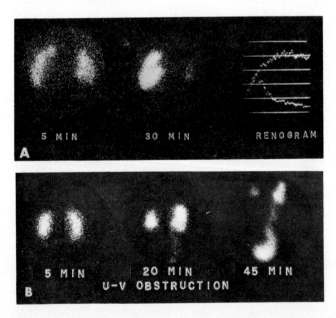

Fig. 9-1. (A) Ureteropelvic obstruction. At 5 min there is prominent defect along medial border of left kidney which is caused by hydronephrotic renal pelvis. At 30 min dilated renal pelvis is noted with retention of radionuclide in left kidney. Obstructive renogram pattern is recorded from that kidney. Nonvisualization of ureter indicates ureteropelvic junction obstruction. (B) Ureterovesical obstruction. Series of images illustrates eventual visualization of entire ureter in obstructive kidney indicating ureterovesical junction obstruction.

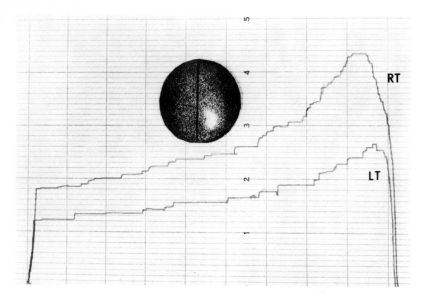

Fig. 9-2. Split crystal technique for deriving renogram curves is not applicable to infant whose entire body is almost encompassed in gamma camera field of vision. "Renogram effect" can be noted on left side due to blood clearance of radionuclide by functioning right kidney. There was no kidney on left side in child. In such cases, regions of interest encompassing only renal areas are necessary for accurate renogram curve derivation.

ever, represents a conglomeration of all of the functional aspects of the normal and/or abnormal kidney. The renogram is too complex a study for casual visual interpretation. As a result, credibility in the renogram was blighted somewhat by the discrepancies observed between the clinical situation and the interpretation.

In the mid-1960s the technique of renogram recording with simultaneous renal imaging using the gamma camera and ^{131}I-Hippuran (12) alleviated many of the earlier technical problems which produced interpretive difficulties. For example, one can correlate an "obstructive" renogram pattern with the scintigram and even localize the site of obstruction (Fig. 9-1A, B). Nonobstructive conditions which mimic an obstructive renogram pattern are easily rejected from diagnostic consideration.

More recently, a further modification of technique involves the use of videotape data-storage devices which enable more accurate localization of renal areas, eliminating unwanted body background activity. This is most important in infants and small children because almost the total body is included within the camera field (Fig. 9-2). A "renogram effect" from blood clearance even in the absence of functioning renal tissue may be observed. One must also be aware of activity in the liver

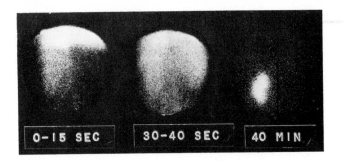

Fig. 9-3. During radionuclide angiography of abdomen, organs which initially appear are kidneys and spleen. Liver does not appear until approximately 15–30 sec following kidneys. This is because primary blood supply to liver is through portal system which circulates through bowel first. One should not confuse liver concentration at 30–40 sec as representing renal tissue. Forty minutes after ^{131}I-Hippuran injection, right kidney is not visualized.

or spleen mimicking renal tissue activity during radionuclide angiographic studies (Fig. 9-3).

The renogram curve, despite its complexity, is still considered a valuable tool because it provides a relative quantitative evaluation of renal function. Standard roentgenographic contrast studies visualize anatomic detail and only imply function in a gross manner.

Renal imaging. Renal imaging with [203]Hg-chlormerodrin received a limited application in pediatric practice primarily because of its relatively large radiation dose to the patient. Mercury-197-chlormerodrin, which has a more reasonable radiation dose, was used routinely for the investigation of renal masses (*13–15*) but hardly replaces roentgenographic techniques which provide the necessary and desired anatomic detail.

Other radiopharmaceuticals, e.g., ^{131}I-Hippuran, which primarily evaluates tubular secretory function, and more recently, ^{99m}Tc-DTPA (*16*), a chelate which evaluates glomerular filtration function, have virtually replaced the mercurials as scanning agents of choice. Improved image quality, resolution, and detail are provided by the more suitable energy range and higher photon flux of the technetium radiopharmaceuticals. In addition, the radiation dose is reduced because of short biological half-lives. Quantification of function can be documented with ^{131}I-Hippuran by the simultaneous derivation of the renogram curves.

Our current technique involves an initial dynamic study with ^{99m}Tc-DTPA recorded on a videotape data-storage device. One can visualize the abdominal aorta and quantitate renal perfusion during the arteriographic phase of the radionuclide study (Fig. 9-4). This technique has been used along with Hippuran renography to accurately predict viability and status of renal transplant recipients. A full discussion of these techniques is beyond the scope and intent of this publication. Delayed

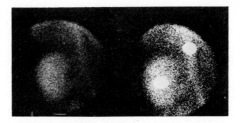

Fig. 9-4. (Left) Radionuclide angiography. During arterial phase of radionuclide angiogram, transplant kidney is visualized as well as abdominal aorta and femoral arteries. Size, contour, and position of kidney is noted. (Right) Regions of interest placed over kidney and aorta (white dots) can record relative perfusion in both areas.

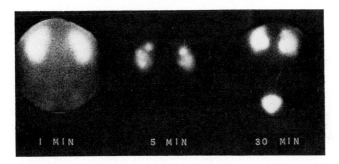

Fig. 9-5. Initial and delayed images with ^{99m}Tc-DTPA. Initially, entire kidney is outlined representing cortex and medullary portions of kidney. By 5 min calices may be individually seen, particularly if there is dilatation of kidney. Renal pelvis and ureter are seen at 30 min.

images with ^{99m}Tc-DTPA can illustrate calyceal, pelvic, ureteral, and bladder structures with considerable detail (Fig. 9-5).

The radionuclide angiogram is followed by an ^{131}I-Hippuran function study with recorded renogram curves. The comparison of renogram curves and low photon flux ^{131}I-Hippuran images with the more detailed ^{99m}Tc-DTPA images increases interpretive accuracy and provides additional information not provided by each study alone. They thus compliment and enhance each other.

Radionuclide cystography. There has been recent interest in the use of radionuclides for the detection of vesicoureteral reflux. The radiation to the gonads from roentgenographic studies has long concerned both the pediatric radiologist and urologist. Such studies are necessary because documentation of reflux is considered to be of prognostic significance. Thus methods to replace the standard roentgenographic techniques were sought.

Theoretically, two methods can be used to detect reflux: the direct and the indirect method. The indirect method (*17, 18*) relies upon the rapid and complete renal clearance of an intravenously injected radio-pharmaceutical. After accumulation in the bladder, probes or a scintillation camera are placed over the upper portions of the renal tracts. As the patient voids, any sudden and significant increase in radioactivity over these areas indicates reflux. The advantages of the indirect method are (A) the bladder is not catheterized, and (B) some assessment of renal function and anatomy can be derived during the early postinjection stage of the study. The indirect method suffers from certain drawbacks. First, the child must cooperate to a considerable degree by retaining bladder urine until adequate renal clearance is achieved, and then the child must void on command. Many children will not or cannot void on command, and younger infants and children will not cooperate at all. Second, vesicoureteral reflux is a dynamic process. Definite and significant reflux occurring during bladder filling may disappear during and after voiding (Fig. 9-6). Such transient but significant reflux into the upper tracts may thus be completely missed by the indirect method. Third, in many of these patients renal function is impaired and considerable activity remains in renal areas. Thus small amounts of reflux may be obscured by this retained activity. The indirect method, therefore, is best suited for those cooperative older children who have adequate renal function.

The direct method (*19–22*) involves catheterization and instillation into the bladder of an appropriate radiopharmaceutical along with normal saline to patient tolerance. Images of the upper tracts to identify reflux are recorded in the posterior and posterior oblique projections (Fig. 9-7). Pre- and post-voiding bladder films may visualize bladder abnormalities. Measurement of the voided urine volume enables the calculation of residual urine volume according to the following formula:

$$\text{Residual volume} = \frac{\text{Voided volume} \times \text{residual count}}{\text{Initial count} - \text{residual count}}.$$

Finally, the drainage time of the upper tract can be quantitated. This value reflects the tonicity of the involved ureter (Fig. 9-8).

A prospective study (*22*) of radionuclide cystography compared with roentgenographic cystography showed the radionuclide method to be more effective in detecting significant vesicoureteral reflux. Of great importance is the marked reduction in radiation dose to the gonads with the radionuclide technique. Approximately 100 radionuclide studies can be performed for each roentgenographic study. Finally, the roentgenographic technique cannot accurately measure residual urine volume and upper tract drainage time—both easily accomplished by the radionuclide technique.

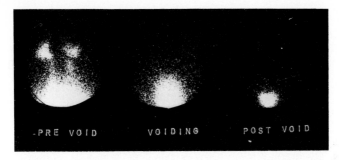

Fig. 9-6. Ureterovesical reflux is dynamic process. Bilateral reflux is seen on prevoiding images. As patient assumed sitting position for voiding, reflux disappeared. Dynamism of reflux has been noted on innumerable occasions. This would indicate that recording of images only during certain phases of examination, such as is done during roentgenographic cystography and indirect radionuclide cystography, may miss number of instances of reflux.

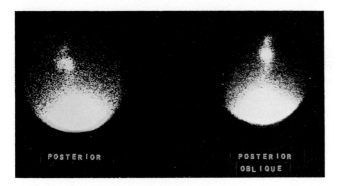

Fig. 9-7. During radionuclide cystography images are initially recorded in posterior and in posterior oblique projections. Note detail which is demonstrable with currently available gamma camera recording instruments.

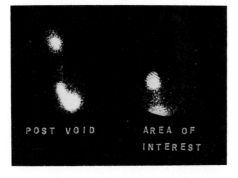

Fig. 9-8. Ureterovesical reflux is demonstrated on left. Area of interest is placed over upper urinary tract. Half-time of radionuclide activity disappearance reflects ureteral tonicity.

Clinical Usefulness

The review of our renography and renal imaging material emphasizes an interesting fact: only about 5% of the studies were completely normal. This is a far smaller percentage of normals than observed with roentgenographic intravenous urography. It would imply that the patient population for radionuclide studies was either highly selected, or, perhaps, the modality is underused at our institution. In any event, the high percentage of abnormal studies has provided a great wealth of material for presentation and discussion. It would be impossible to illustrate the indications and the clinical usefulness of all of these studies, and therefore we have attempted to categorize those recurrent conditions in which renography and renal imaging are most useful.

Allergy to contrast material. Although sensitivity to iodinated contrast material is somewhat unusual in infants and children, the possibility of such a reaction always dictates an awareness of its occurrence and an immediate therapeutic response. Whenever a history of previous reaction is elicited, several steps are undertaken before the examination. A thorough history and documentation of the previous reaction is of paramount importance. The necessity for examination is carefully weighed by the attending physician and the radiologist. If the examination is warranted and deemed necessary, then an allergist is consulted along with an anesthesiologist. Premedication with antihistamines and corticosteroids is decided individually in each case. In spite of these precautions, such an examination is performed with much concern and trepidation. A thorough discussion with the parents is mandatory, and a written consent is considered appropriate.

In these problem cases, the determination of renal function can be readily accomplished with renography and renal imaging. To our knowledge, there has never been reported a reaction to a radioiodinated radiopharmaceutical for renal studies. This is probably because the number of molecules of radioactive iodine is infinitesimally small compared with roentgenographic studies. Indeed, it has often been stated that the number of iodine molecules present in a renogram study is less than that received from the normal daily dietary iodinated salt intake. Likewise, reactions to ^{99m}Tc-labeled renal agents have not been reported.

Parental consent. In some instances, the parents will refuse to permit a roentgenographic exam but will accept renography and radionuclide imaging. It should be pointed out that both modalities rely upon the use of ionizing radiation. The absorbed radiation from radionuclide studies, however, is lower than comparable roentgenographic studies.

Poor renal function. The quality of roentgenographic studies deteriorates directly with decreasing renal function. As a result, the worst studies are recorded in those patients that need them most. An elevated blood urea nitrogen portends a poor roentgenographic visualization, and,

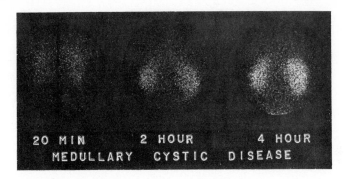

Fig. 9-9. Delayed ^{99m}Tc-DTPA images indicate kidney size, position, and evident diminished renal function in patient with medullary cystic disease. Blood urea nitrogen level at time of examination was 120. Visualization of urinary tracts could not be achieved with roentgenographic techniques.

indeed, double dose, drip infusion, and tomographic techniques are advocated routinely in such patients.

Visualization of the kidneys can often be accomplished with radionuclide imaging in spite of nonvisualization during intravenous urography. Information about renal position, size, and function can be obtained even in patients with a blood urea nitrogen well over 100 (Fig. 9-9).

Nonvisualization of a kidney. In addition to those instances when intravenous urography is performed for direct evidence of renal disease, renal abnormalities are frequently found during screening examinations. For example, all patients receiving contrast material during cardiac catherization or neuroradiological studies are also examined with a roentgenogram of the abdomen. A significant incidence of nonvisualization of a kidney has been noted. Congenital absence of a kidney, however, is uncommon. Documentation of the etiology for nonvisualization of a kidney is important for patient management. Cystoscopy will often demonstrate the presence of a ureter and angiography has been advocated to demonstrate the presence of a renal artery. Cystoscopy, particularly of male infants in the newborn period, requires expertise and extreme care. Angiography in an otherwise asymptomatic individual is difficult to justify.

Radionuclide imaging readily resolves these problems and on numerous occasions an ectopic kidney location (Fig. 9-10A, B) has been documented. Delayed renal images will often illustrate those extremely poorly functioning renal elements which are overlooked on intravenous urography. The absence of an evident vascular blush during radionuclide angiography or delayed accumulation of radionuclide in a functioning

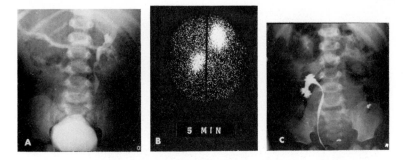

Fig. 9-10. (A) Left kidney could not be visualized in spite of multiple projections on two examinations. (B) Radionuclide image with ^{131}I-Hippuran readily demonstrates ectopic pelvic location of kidney which was further documented during C, a retrograde pyelogram.

renal element warrants a diagnosis of absent renal tissue and cystoscopy and angiography can be delayed to a more appropriate time.

The value of radionuclide imaging to detect the presence and function of the kidneys in children with bilateral nonvisualization on intravenous urography has also been proved on many occasions. Lack of preparation, gas within the bowel, and poor concentration of the contrast material due to hydration are causes of inadequate visualization of the kidneys during intravenous urography. In some instances, double doses or rescheduling following additional preparation may prove futile. Renography and renal imaging will often provide the necessary information without further preparation.

Unilateral renal masses in the new born. A flank mass in a neonate provides considerable concern for the practicing pediatrician. The most common causes for such a mass are (A) unilateral multicystic kidney; (B) unilateral hydronephrosis; (C) hamartoma of the kidney; and (D) renal vein thrombosis. Therapy for each of these lesions varies. It therefore behooves the surgeon to characterize the lesion preoperatively.

Clinically, renal vein thrombosis is frequently noted in infants of diabetic mothers or following dehydration (from whatever cause). It appears with a flank mass and hematuria. The kidney may or may not be visualized on an intravenous urogram and is usually enlarged. The diagnosis is difficult and may even require renal vein catherization for visualization of a thrombus.

Neoplasms of the kidney are uncommon in the new-born period. The most frequent lesion is a hamartoma of the kidney (23). This has often been described as a neonatal Wilms' tumor. The hamartoma is more benign than the Wilms' tumor. Again, it is most difficult to diagnose and requires histology for confirmation. We have had insufficient experience

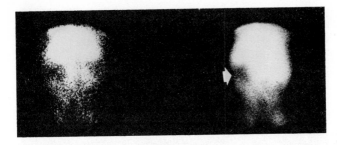

Fig. 9-11. (Left) Unilateral multicystic kidney presents as relatively avascular lesion during radionuclide angiography with ^{99m}Tc-DTPA. (Right) Absence of function within unilateral multicystic kidney persists on delayed images.

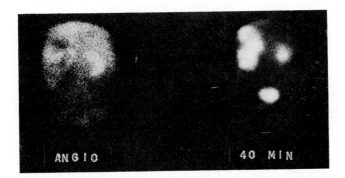

Fig. 9-12. Hydronephrosis may also be visualized as avascular mass during angiogram portion (left) of study. But evidence of function is always noted on delayed images (right) which readily distinguishes it from multicystic kidney. Delayed images must be obtained for periods up to 24 hr when function is minimal.

with radionuclide imaging of such lesions to warrant describing a characteristic appearance.

The most commonly encountered renal flank masses are the unilateral multicystic kidney and unilateral hydronephrosis. The incidence varies depending upon the reporting institution. At our institution, which is primarily a referral center, the unilateral multicystic kidney is more commonly observed. These two lesions which comprise the bulk of neonatal renal masses in our experience are readily differentiated with radionuclide angiography and renal imaging. The cystic nature of the unilateral multicystic kidney produces a region of decreased radionuclide activity during radionuclide angiography (Fig. 9-11). This locus of decreased radionuclide activity persists, and little if any accumulation of ^{131}I-Hippuran will be noted even on delayed images up to 24 hr. Hydronephrosis, on the other hand, may also be visualized initially as an avascular lesion, but the accumulation of radionuclide within the

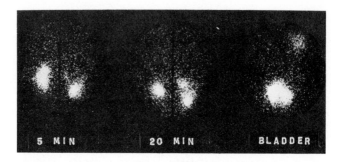

Fig. 9-13. Duplicate kidney segment. Recurrent urinary tract infections led to examination. Upper pole of right kidney exhibits poor function at 5 min with ^{131}I-Hippuran. At 20 min, however, evident function appears. Bladder study shows retention within upper pole duplication. Small defect at base of bladder represents ureterocoele of duplicated kidney.

hydronephrotic pelvis secondary to minimal renal function is noted in almost every case (Fig. 9-12). This has been observed even when inadequate or nonvisualization of the hydronephrotic kidney on delayed intravenous urography has occurred.

Estimation of local function. It is necessary on occasion to surgically remove abnormal portions of the urinary tract when function is minimal, and there is little chance of recovery in spite of treatment. One often resects a portion of the kidney when a duplication exists. This is particularly so when infection is recurrent in the duplicated segment. It is difficult to evaluate the degree of function by intravenous urography and only a visual estimate can be achieved. Renography and renal imaging is much more useful for quantitating the degree of function (Fig. 9-13). Thus radionuclide studies are recommended for those patients who are considered for surgical resection of a portion or all of the functioning renal unit.

Since renography can quantitate the degree of function remaining in a renal unit, it is also of value in medical management. Long-term prospective studies, e.g., following relief of unilateral obstruction and hydronephrosis, may perhaps dictate the efficacy of surgical as well as medical management and indicate prognostic or therapeutic criteria for salvage versus resection of the hydronephrotic element.

Trauma. The ease of performance and safety of nuclear renal imaging has given these techniques an important role in the diagnosis of renal lacerations and fractures due to trauma. In patients not deemed candidates for contrast angiography, radionuclide studies may provide diagnostic information (Fig. 9-14).

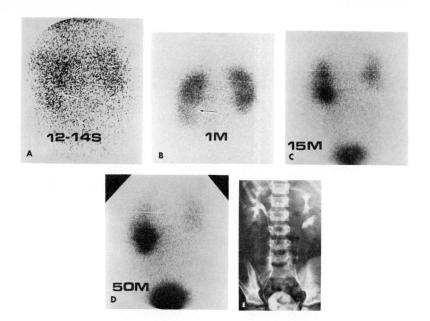

Fig. 9-14. Trauma. Patient was playing football when struck in left flank. He developed hematuria. (A) ^{99m}Tc-DTPA scintiphoto (12–14 sec after injection) shows normal kidney on right and elongated left kidney with decreased perfusion to medial portion of lower pole (arrow). (B) Later scintiphoto (1 min) reveals normal right kidney and decreased activity in medial portion of left lower pole (arrow). (C) 15 min later scintiphoto shows marked increase in activity, as material is excreted, in region of perfusion defect. (D) 50-min scintiphoto shows persistence of left lower pole accumulation while remainder of material has passed to bladder, suggesting extravasation of urine in a collection (urinoma). (E) Intravenous pyelogram (15-min film) confirms collection (left kidney on reader's right). (Study courtesy of David L. Gilday, The Hospital for Sick Children, Toronto.)

Summary

An attempt has been made to define the definitive indications for the use of renal imaging, renography, and radionuclide cystography in childhood. Limitations of space prohibit a comprehensive discussion of all of the criteria for such studies. The more common indications and uses are discussed. It is of importance to recognize the simplicity of these examinations which require no preparation, offer a minimum morbidity to the child, and in most instances produce less radiation burden than comparable roentgenographic techniques. The potential for research in the field of pediatric urology with such techniques is unlimited. Recognition of the usefulness of nuclear medicine techniques by the pediatrician and practicing clinician will increase as these studies become more available.

Acknowledgments

The authors wish to express gratitude to Mildred Early, Roxann Stawicki, and Sue Weiss for their able technological assistance and to Joanne Sedlmeir for her editorial assistance in the preparation of this manuscript.

References

1. DECKART VON H: Nuklearmedizinische nephrologische Untersuchungsverfahren in der Pädiatrie. *Kinderaerztl Prax* 34: 197–205, 1966

2. GOLDMAN HS, FREEMAN LM: Radiographic and radioisotopic methods of evaluation of the kidneys and urinary tract. *Pediatr Clin North Am* 18: 409–434, 1971

3. KATHEL BL: Radioisotope renography as a renal function test in the newborn. *Arch Dis Child* 46: 314–320, 1971

4. LEFCOE S, NOGRADY MB, ROSENTHALL L: Radionuclide scanning complementing high dose urography in children. *J Can Assoc Radiol* 21: 266–269, 1970

5. MAY P, BERBERICH R, BURWICK P, et al: Die Bedeutung seitengetrennter Isotopen-Clearance Untersuchungen für die Indikation zu kinderurologischen Eingraffen. *Urologe* 10: 201–205, 1971

6. MUSSA GC, MAURI MM, BACOLLA D: Utilita della scintigrafia renale a colori in patologia pediatrica. *Minerva Pediatr* 22: 335–349, 1970

7. RADWIN HM, NOVOSELSKY SP: The gamma camera in pediatric urologic diagnosis. *J Urol* 97: 942–947, 1967

8. SHULER SE, MECKSTROTH GR, MAXFIELD WS: Scintillation camera in pediatric renal disease. *Am J Dis Child* 120: 115–122, 1970

9. WINTER CC: Pediatric urological tests using radioisotopes. *J Urol* 95: 584–587, 1966

10. TAPLIN BV, MEREDITH OM, KADE H, et al: The radioisotope renogram. *J Lab Clin Med* 48: 886, 1956

11. WINTER CC: A clinical study of a new renal function test. *J Urol* 76: 182, 1956

12. BURKE G, HALKO A, COE FL: Dynamic clinical studies with radioisotopes and the scintillation camera. *JAMA* 197: 85–94, 1966

13. MUSSA GC, MAURI MM, BACOLLA D: Scintiscans with ^{197}Hg labelled chlormerodrin in the diagnosis of renal tumors and congenital deformities in infants. *Panminerva Med* 13: 394–403, 1971

14. REISNER S, LUBIN E, STARK H, et al: The use of renal scanning in the investigation of flank masses in the neonatal period. *Helv Paediatr Acta* 26: 39–45, 1971

15. SAMUELS LD: Scans in children with renal tumors. *J Urol* 107: 127–132, 1972

16. HAUSER W, ATKINS HL, NELSON KG, et al: Technetium-^{99m}DTPA: A new radiopharmaceutical for brain and kidney scanning. *Radiology* 94: 679–684, 1970

17. DODGE AE: Vesicoureteric reflux. *Lancet* 1: 303–304, 1963

18. HANDMAKER H, McRAE J, BUCK EG: Intravenous radionuclide voiding cystography (IRVC). *Radiology* 108: 703–705, 1973

19. WINTER CC: New test for vesicoureteral reflux: an external technique using radioisotopes. *J Urol* 81: 105–111, 1959

20. CORRIERE JN, KUHL DE, MURPHY JJ: The Use of [99mTc] labeled sulfur colloid to study particle dynamics in the urinary tract. *Invest Urol* 4: 570–575, 1967

21. BLAUFOX MD, GRUSKIN A, SANDLER P, et al: Radionuclide scintigraphy for detection of vesicoureteral reflux in children. *J Pediatr* 79: 239–247, 1971

22. CONWAY JJ, KING LR, BELMAN AB, et al: Detection of vesicoureteral reflux with radionuclide cystography. *Am J Roentgenol Radium Ther Nucl Med* 115: 720–727, 1972

23. BERDON WE, WIGGER HJ, BAKER RH: Fetal renal hamartoma—A benign tumor to be distinguished from Wilm's tumor. *Am J Roentgenol Radium Ther Nucl Med* 118: 18–27, 1973

Discussion

Peter E. Valk (Donner Laboratory, Berkeley, Calif): Why do you use ^{131}I-hippurate for anatomical studies of the kidneys, ureters, and bladder rather than using one of the ^{99m}Tc compounds which are excreted in the urine and retained by the renal cortex?

Dr. Conway: I have used those compounds which are readily commercially available to me in my practice. I do not have access to many products which are available in many university centers. Only recently have ^{99m}Tc-chelate radiopharmaceuticals been made available. With the advent of ^{99m}Tc-labeled chelates, I now have preference for anatomic studies with ^{99m}Tc. One still must use Hippuran for function evaluation.

Daniel Schere (Children's Hospital, Buenos Aires, Argentina): How many false negatives do you get with radionuclide cystography?

Dr. Conway: The earlier prospective clinical study comparing radionuclide cystography with roentgenographic cystography showed as many examples of reflux that were missed with radionuclide cystography as were missed with roentgenographic cystography. However, approximately one half of these misses were examples of transient distal ureteral reflux which are considered to be of no significance. Indeed, this type of reflux may be an artifact of the technique. With better techniques that have been developed in radionuclide cystography and the higher resolution of the HP gamma camera system, it is concluded that the radionuclide technique is much more sensitive than the roentgenographic technique for detecting significant vesicoureteral reflux.

Chapter **10**

Bone

Edward G. Bell and David F. Mahon

D espite the excellent resolution of skeletal detail that is provided by x-ray studies, there are certain shortcomings that explain the continuing interest in other diagnostic modes for investigation of bone. X-ray examination cannot distinguish differences in bone density before decreases of 30–50% in bone calcium have occurred. Yet many diseases in their early or advanced stages involve changes of lesser magnitude.

Bone Seeking Radiopharmaceuticals

The use of radioactive labels attached to bone seeking substances has been the subject of investigation for many years. It was appreciated early that this was a fruitful line of investigation and presumably would reflect not only on the structure of bone but on the function of the skeleton. The earliest available bone seeking radionuclides, ^{32}P and ^{45}Ca were limited in clinical application because their in vivo distribution could not be adequately measured by external radiation detectors. In 1942 Treadwell evaluated ^{85}Sr and found that the radionuclide accumulated in metastases from breast and prostate malignancies. He measured the uptake of ^{85}Sr in abnormal bone by use of an external probe moved over the skeleton.

A rather large number of substances are taken up in bone; these are listed in Table 10-1 (1). While some of these substances are normal constituents of bone and their uptake reflects normal concentrating mechanisms, others are not normally found and are accumulated as a result of

TABLE 10-1. Bone Seeking Substances (Ref *1*.)

Classification	Elements
Alkaline earth metals	Be, Mg, Ca, Sr, Ba, Ra
Aluminum metals	Ga, In
Transition metals	Sc, Y, La
Lanthanides	Lu, Er, Sm, Dy
Actinides	Uranyl ion
Group IVB metals	Sn, Pb
Group IVA metals	Zr, Hf
Group VB metals	Bi
Group VIA transition metals	W
Halogens	F
Compounds	Alizarin, tetracycline, Tc-Sn polyphosphate, pyrophosphate, or diphosphonate compounds

their being normal analogs for physiological substances (*2, 3*). Or they accumulate on bone because they are bound to physiological carriers or to the surface of bone. Strontium is an example of the former and the technetium complexes of the latter.

All of these bone seeking radionuclides reach the bone by the blood supply. One mechanism of increased accumulation at disease sites may be the increased vascularity at these locations (*4*). While increased vasculature may not be the entire explanation, it is known that in most disease entities where there is an increased accretion of the bone-seeker there is an increased bone blood flow.

While not yet proven by definitive experiment, it is suggested that initially the bone seeking radiopharmaceutical is adsorbed on the surface of bone. This is independent of the chemical nature of the material, is dependent only on blood flow, and is relatively rapid. The second kinetic step involves the heteroionic exchange between the bone-seekers and the normal osseous ionic constituents; this is also relatively rapid and is indirectly related to bone blood flow. The third step is diffusion of the tracer within the bone tissue; this is a relatively slow kinetic step and is not of practical consideration when imaging the skeleton with the newer short-lived ^{99m}Tc-labeled bone seeking radiopharmaceuticals.

Of the group of bone-seekers shown in Table 10-1 there are four which have been used in adult clinical nuclear medicine; these are listed with their physical properties in Table 10-2. It is helpful to consider their characteristics to see why they are not all useful in the pediatric age group.

The two isotopes of strontium are analogs of calcium and concentrate in the mineral phase of bone. The retention of strontium within bone may be described by a multiexponential equation having the three components described earlier. It has been shown that the pediatric age group has a higher fraction of the slowest third phase than do older people. Strontium-85 accumulates in bony lesions and produces moderately satisfactory bone scans 3–7 days after the injection of the nitrate salt. The long half-life is associated with a high radiation dose; accordingly, the nuclide is restricted to use in patients with documented malignancies. It is not licensed for use in children or for use in adults with benign disease.

Strontium-87m results in a radiation dose less than 1% of the dose associated with ^{85}Sr. It may be used in studying benign disease even in children. Its half-life is too short and the blood clearance too slow; therefore, by the time one has to wait for the extraosseous activity to decrease, there are too few photons remaining for satisfactory imaging.

Fluorine-18 is an excellent bone imaging agent (5). It may be administered orally or intravenously with approximately 50% of the administered dose localizing in bone and the remainder cleared rapidly by the kidneys. The short half-life confers a low radiation dose. It may be safely used in studying malignant and benign bone disorders in children. The high-energy photons associated with the decay of ^{18}F are far from ideal for the scintillation camera because of the low detection sensitivity. In addition, the short half-life poses a significant supply problem because it requires close geographic proximity to the source of production.

Technetium-99m in the pertechnetate form is not a bone-seeker, and it is not satisfactory for detecting bone lesions (6). However, it has been found that when ^{99m}Tc is complexed with tin and a compound of phosphorous such as polyphosphate (7), pyrophosphate (8), or diphosphonate (9) a highly specific bone seeking tracer results. The compounds are easily prepared by a single kit method at minimal cost and deliver relatively low radiation doses. The ^{99m}Tc compounds may be safely used to study both benign and malignant bone disease in children and are the preferred agents available today. These factors now place bone scanning

TABLE 10-2. Properties of Clinically Useful Bone–Seekers

Nuclide	Half-life	Gamma emission (keV)	Avg. skeletal dose (rads)	Usual administered adult dose
^{85}Sr	65 days	514	3.1/100 μCi	100 μCi
^{87m}Sr	2.7 hr	388	0.13/1 mCi	1–4 mCi
^{18}F (5)	1.85 hr	511 (annihilation)	0.18/1 mCi	1–5 mCi
^{99m}TcPP (7), HEDPA (9), Methylene diphosphonate (15), pyrophosphate (8)	6 hr	140	0.05/1 mCi	10–15 mCi

in the pediatric age group within the reach of even modest nuclear medicine facilities.

The Growing Skeleton

There are marked differences between the skeletal activity of young growing animals and nongrowing adults. An increasing body of evidence indicates that as the skeleton matures, a smaller and smaller fraction of the bone remains in equilibrium with the body fluids. It has also been shown that the growing bone has a higher level of hydration than the adult compact bone. Thus materials from the plasma may both reach and be removed from the growing bone at a faster rate than that associated with adult bone. Experimental evidence exists that both the deposition and mobilization of intravenously administered bone-seekers vary directly with the growth rate of the bone. Comar (10) and Bauer (11) showed that the ratio of the specific activities of diaphyseal bone to that of epiphyseal bone rose continually from a value below unity to a value above unity over a period of approximately 60 days after the administration of ^{45}Ca in pigs and rats. This change in the ratio reflected the high initial activity in the epiphyseal center followed by a rapid loss with time whereas the diaphyseal area remained essentially constant.

This dynamic equilibrium between bone and its blood supply involves the continuous deposition of Ca^{2+}, PO_4^{3-}, and other trace ions in the bone mineral pool. This localized effect in certain growth areas of the

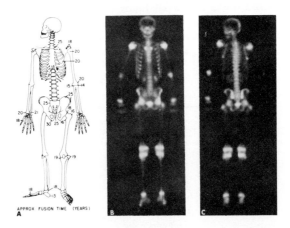

Fig. 10-1. Normal scan and average closure time for epiphyseal growth centers. A illustrates average epiphyseal closure time in years for both females and males. B and C are total-body scans in anterior and posterior projections of 14-year-old boy obtained with ^{99m}Tc-diphosphonate. Study is within normal limits. Note avid accumulation in epiphyseal growth centers.

normal skeleton of the growing child leads to a lack of homogeneity in the physicochemical composition of bone mineral. Thus the injection of radioactive bone seekers will lead to a nonuniform distribution of the radionuclide in direct response to the localized bone activity. This phenomenon is reflected in the bone scan of a normal, growing child as striking areas of accumulation in the epiphyseal growth centers.

The distribution of radioactivity in the skeleton of the growing child is age-dependent and these epiphyseal concentrations decrease as bone growth decreases. Figure 10-1 illustrates the total-body scan obtained with ^{99m}Tc-diphosphonate in a 14-year-old boy. The scans are compared with a skeleton illustrating the average time in years for cessation of growth in several growth centers.

Calculation of the Administered Dose

It is the authors' feeling that the dose should be administered on the basis of surface area in that this more accurately reflects metabolic activity (12). It has been shown that surface area may be approximated as a power function of the body weight (13); the detailed calculations are not of value for the reader and thus will not be described here. The results of the calculations are shown in Appendix Tables A-2 and A-3. Tables A-2 and A-3 list the body weight in kilograms and pounds respectively, calculated surface area, and the resultant dose factor. The dose factor is the multiplier for the usual adult dose. For example, if the child's weight is 20 kg and the usual adult dose is 15 mCi of the ^{99m}Tc compound, the child's dose is 0.44×15 mCi $= 6.6$ mCi.

The child's weight is recorded in the hospital chart in either pounds or kilograms depending upon the pediatric practice in varying hospitals. In the authors' department graphs are posted in the Radiopharmaceutical Laboratory and are available immediately for the technical staff to calculate the doses for any of the pediatric radioisotopic examinations.

Performing the Scan

It is the authors' belief that there is a definite need to image the entire body to properly assess the skeleton for unusual or abnormal areas of accretion of the radiopharmaceutical. This may be done with a rectilinear scanner or, preferably, with the total-body scanning attachments presently available for scintillation cameras.

Following the total-body image, the scintillation camera is used to obtain four views of the head (not available on the total-body scan) and selected views of areas of interest. The areas of interest represent either abnormal or suspicious areas demonstrated on the total-body scan or areas which are clinically suspected. In small children or infants, our practice is to use the converging collimator and in certain particular cases the pinhole collimator for the selected camera images. In larger children, we use a parallel-hole collimator and occasionally the pinhole collimator for the selected static images.

It must be emphasized that there is no single routine for the performance of all bone scans after a total-body image is obtained. For example, if the child complains of hip pain, then every effort should be made to prove definitely that there is no evidence for areas of either increased or decreased uptake. It is usually assuring to image the hip joints bilaterally in the anterior, posterior, and anterior oblique projections and also anteriorly with the leg in maximum internal rotation. These multiple images may be easily obtained in logistically feasible times with the ^{99m}Tc-labeled bone-seekers and the scintillation camera.

The Abnormal Bone Scan

In the interpretation of bone images, each part of the skeleton is compared with both the contralateral side and also the adjacent area. If there is a significant localized increase in the bone blood flow, there will be an abnormally high deposition of the agent in that site. Abnormal accumulation may be seen with either primary or secondary tumors, collagen diseases, infectious diseases, recent fractures, and skeletal manifestations of generalized pediatric diseases.

Lesions which lead to a decrease in localized bone blood flow have decreased accretion of the bone-seekers. Before the advent of the ^{99m}Tc-labeled compounds, these were not generally visualized on bone scanning; now with the use of high-resolution collimators it is possible to detect these lesions. It was only five years ago that Bell, et al (14) described asymmetrical areas of radiation as being the only detectable cause of decreased accumulation of the bone-seekers. Today, abnormal scans, with the involved area having a decrease in the concentration of the radiopharmaceutical as compared to the adjacent area, have been seen with recent aseptic necrosis of the femoral head, solitary bone cysts, some cases of histiocytosis-X, and rare cases of nearly total replacement of bone by fast-growing metastatic disease in addition to asymmetrical fields of external radiation.

Some selected points in clinical interpretation are described by review of the following descriptive figures. The pathologies illustrated are osteogenic sarcoma, osteoid osteoma, synovial sarcoma, neuroblastoma, aneurysmal bone cyst, acute osteomyelitis, cellulitis, acute rheumatic fever, trauma, traumatic synovitis, and aseptic necrosis of the femoral head.

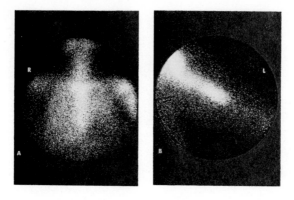

Fig. 10-2. Osteogenic sarcoma of left humerus obtained (A) with diverging collimator, 50,000 counts in 55 sec. and (B) with pinhole collimator, 100,000 counts in 300 sec.

Figure 10-2 illustrates *osteogenic sarcoma* in a 17-year-old girl with 1-month history of swelling of left shoulder and proximal left humerus. The study was performed with 15 mCi of ^{99m}Tc-polyphosphate. The image on the right represents a scan of the anterior thorax obtained with the pinhole collimator; the image has 100,000 counts and took 300 sec. While the quality is poor, it does allow one to compare the area scanned for abnormal or suspicious areas of increased accumulation of the radiopharmaceutical. The image on the left represents an anterior image of the proximal aspect of the left humerus using the diverging collimator (50,000 in 55 sec). The abnormal accumulation is noted in the humeral head and proximal third of the humeral shaft. The examination of the specimen following a forequarter amputation showed osteogenic sarcoma of the humerus with extension into muscle and soft tissue but not through the shoulder joint capsule. The tumor measured $9 \times 7 \times 7$ cm; it extended from the shaft through the epiphysis into the head of the humerus.

In our experience, the avidity of *osteoid osteomas* for bone seeking radiopharmaceuticals is variable. It is our practice to grade the uptake in the lesion with respect to the urinary bladder concentration. The lesions which accumulate the radiopharmaceutical equal to the bladder are classed Grade 4 (4/4); those lesions which are just visible above normal bone are classed Grade 1 (1/4). Those lesions which accrete the agents to a lesser extent than normal bone are merely classified as void areas. These points are illustrated in Fig. 10-3. Figure 10-3A is a 4-year-old girl with right hip pain. The x-ray films revealed sclerotic changes surrounding two cystic rarefactions; there was no periosteal new bone. The anterior pelvis bone scan obtained with 6.7 mCi ^{99m}Tc-polyphos-

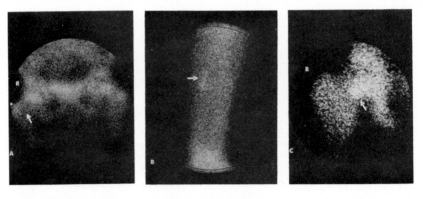

Fig. 10-3. Osteoid osteoma. (A) Old healing osteoid osteoma in femoral neck; area is void of uptake. (B) Osteoid osteoma in ulna; uptake graded 1/4. (C) Osteoid osteoma in femoral neck; uptake graded 3/4 (provided by H. Handmaker).

phate illustrated decreased uptake in the femoral neck; the femoral-head growth center appeared normal. The pathological examination revealed an old healing osteoid osteoma with sclerotic bone fragments. Figure 10-3B is an image obtained with 15 mCi ^{99m}Tc-polyphosphate of the left forearm of a young lady with pain in the midshaft of her ulna. The quality of uptake was graded 1 (1/4); the pathological examination revealed an osteoid osteoma. Figure 10-3C shows a lesion in the right femoral neck of a pediatric patient; the lesion was graded 3 (3/4). An osteoid osteoma was found at surgery.

Figure 10-4 shows a *synovial sarcoma* in a 17-year-old boy with a lump in his left wrist for over 1 year. One week before the scan he suffered trauma to the wrist and noted swelling and pain in the area. X-ray films of the region illustrated a soft-tissue mass arising between the ulna and radius. It involved the bone in a secondary fashion causing

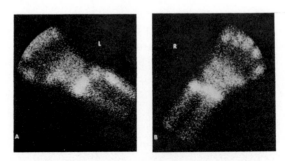

Fig. 10-4. Synovial sarcoma of left forearm (A) and normal right side (B).

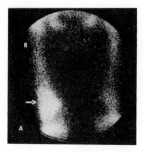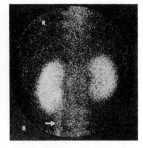

Fig. 10-5. Neuroblastoma (A) showing avid uptake in metastatic disease in right femur. Neuroblastoma (B) showing decreased uptake in metastatic disease of lumbar spine. Note activity in right ureter due to obstructive uropathy (arrow).

separation, thinning, and interference with growth. The bone scan was performed with 15 mCi of ^{99m}Tc-diphosphonate; 25,000 in 30 sec. The bone scan (Fig. 10-4A) shows deformity in the distal portion of the left ulna, decreased accumulation in the growth plate, and increased activity extending proximally along the ulnar shaft. The pathological evaluation of the specimen revealed a synovial sarcoma arising between the ulna and radius. There was periosteal new bone formation on the radial side of the ulna. The bone was not invaded by the malignant tissue.

Several patients with *neuroblastomas* have had metastatic disease to the skeleton demonstrated by bone scanning. Figure 10-5A is the bone scan in a 1-year-old boy with known neuroblastoma. A marked abnormal increased accumulation is noted in the distal aspect of the right femur. This area was shown to be involved with the tumor at the time of autopsy. Figure 10-5B shows the lumbar spine in a 15-year-old boy with known neuroblastoma. The x-ray films were normal. At time of autopsy, diffuse and extensive involvement of the lumbar spine by the primary disease was noted. Close inspection of the bone scan reveals that the uptake in upper lumbar spine is diffusely decreased below what is normally noted (compare with the renal activity). While the scan is abnormal, the presence of a widespread and diffuse decrease in uptake is more difficult to assess than localized areas of increased uptake. As a point of comparison, it is noteworthy to remind the reader that occasionally in diffuse metastatic disease from a breast primary in the adult female there is diffuse *increased* uptake of the bone-seeker in the vertebral column. These cases are also more difficult to assess than cases of localized increased uptake. Note also the activity in the ureter arising from the right kidney (arrow). Obstruction in the urinary outflow tract may be detected by use of the ^{99m}Tc-labeled bone-seekers or ^{18}F-sodium fluoride.

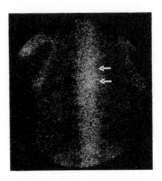

Fig. 10-6. Aneurysmal bone cyst (arrows) of thoracic spine.

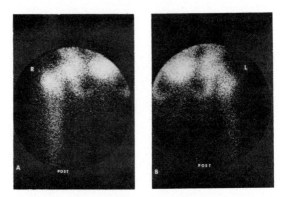

Fig. 10-7. Acute osteomyelitis of right
hip (A). Left side (B) is normal.

Figure 10-6 shows an *aneurysmal bone* cyst in a 13-year-old girl with tingling and numbness in lower extremities 2 weeks after a blow to her vertex while diving in shallow water. The x-ray tomographic films revealed changes in the transverse pedicle and lamina posteriorly and irregular trabecula anteriorly consistent with a benign tumor of bone. The image shown here was obtained with ^{99m}Tc-polyphosphate using the diverging collimator. The study is abnormal and illustrates subtle accumulation in the sixth thoracic vertebral body and to a lesser extent in the fifth vertebral body (arrows). The accumulation was graded 1 (1/4). An aneurysmal bone cyst in the thoracic spine at the level of the sixth vertebral body with superior extension was found at surgery.

Acute osteomyelitis in a 6-year-old girl with acute onset of fever and right leg pain is shown in Fig. 10-7. On the day of bone scan, the right hip was extremely tender to palpation with marked limitation of passive movement. The x-ray films were negative. The blood culture was positive for staphylococcus aureus. The study was performed with 6.6 mCi ^{99m}Tc-polyphosphate. The abnormality, Grade 2 (2/4), is seen in the trochanteric region of the right femur. The x-ray films became abnormal 2 weeks later. The acute osteomyelitis was successfully treated with the appropriate antibiotic.

Soft-tissue inflammatory disease may give rise to abnormal bone scans and thus may be confused with osteomyelitis or other bone diseases. Figure 10-8 gives the study obtained in an 8-year-old girl who had a Wilms' tumor of the left kidney removed 2 weeks before the first scan. She was treated with actinomycin-D following surgery, through an intravenous cut-down in her left ankle. At the time of the first scan she had superficial pain and erythematous changes in her left foot and in the anterior aspect of the left lower limb. The scans were performed with 7.5 mCi ^{99m}Tc-polyphosphate. Figure 10-8A, the first study at 2 weeks post surgery, shows increased uptake in the left foot, tibia, and to a lesser extent the epiphyseal growth centers at the knee. It was felt that hypervascularity related to soft-tissue inflammation was the most probable explanation; however, osteomyelitis could not be excluded. The probability of metastatic disease from the Wilms' primary was remote and would not lead to the signs of hypervascularity. The patient was treated with antibiotics. The second study, Fig. 10-8B at 7 weeks, showed increased uptake in the left foot and left knee with resolution of the previously noted uptake in the left tibia. Antibiotics were discontinued. The last study, Fig. 10-8C at 14 weeks, was interpreted as being within normal limits. While osteomyelitis could not be excluded as being a contributor to the abnormal series, it is felt that the major factor was cellu-

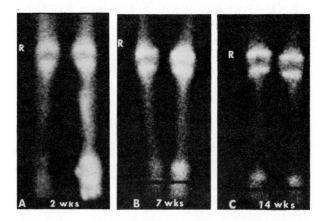

Fig. 10-8. Cellulitis (A) lower limbs (knees to feet) 2 weeks post surgery, (B) 7 weeks post surgery, and (C) 14 weeks post surgery.

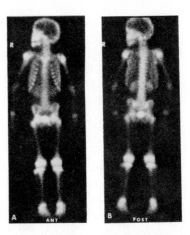

Fig. 10-9. Acute rheumatic fever. Total-body scan anterior (A) and posterior (B). There is no evidence of disease.

litis and phlebitis related to the intravenous therapy the patient was receiving as partial systemic treatment for her Wilms' tumor.

In our experience to date, *acute rheumatic fever* has yielded negative bone scans. The importance of the bone scan lies in excluding acute osteomyelitis or juvenile rheumatoid arthritis. In our limited experience, septic arthritis also yields negative bone scans and thus may not be differentiated from acute rheumatic fever by this diagnostic modality. Whether this proves to be a consistent finding may be determined only by additional experience. Figure 10-9 is the study obtained in a 6-year-old boy who presented with right leg pain, swelling, erythema, and tenderness of right knee and right ankle. He then developed swelling and erythema of his left knee and ankle. The bone scan was performed with 7.1 mCi of ^{99m}Tc-diphosphonate. The total-body scans were interpreted as being within normal limits and were thus compatible with acute rheumatic fever. The diagnosis was confirmed subsequently by routine clinical tests.

Fractures generally are within normal limits on bone scanning within 1–3 days following the trauma unless there is marked bony destruction. The scan then becomes abnormal with the lesion accreting the radiopharmaceutical at variable levels (grade 1/4 to grade 4/4). The fracture site commonly returns to normal levels at time periods from 6 to 12 months following the trauma. Figure 10-10 shows trauma in a young girl who was involved in an automobile accident and suffered a dislocated right hip and injury to left knee. The x-ray films of the left knee showed a fluid-fat level with no evidence of a fracture. The bone scan was performed with 15 mCi ^{99m}Tc-diphosphonate with the anterior view of the knees obtained with a diverging collimator. Diffuse increased uptake is

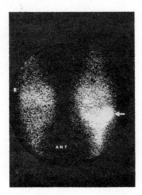

Fig. 10-10.   Fracture of left lateral tibial condyle (arrow).

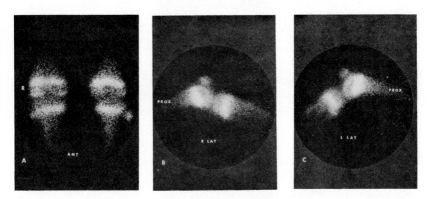

Fig. 10-11.   Traumatic synovitis of left knee (A) anterior,
(B) right lateral, and (C) left lateral. Images are normal.

noted in the proximal aspect of the left tibia with an avid area, Grade 4
(4/4), in the lateral tibial condyle. This was interpreted as a fracture (in
view of the history of trauma). A repeat x-ray film demonstrated the
fracture in the left lateral tibial condyle.

Figure 10-11 is the study obtained in a 7-year-old boy who
awakened 7 days before this study with right knee pain on weight-bear-
ing and some stiffness. He developed an effusion which was blood tinged;
it supported no growth on culture. The x-ray films were negative. The
clinical diagnosis was either *traumatic synovitis* or acute osteomyelitis.
The bone scan was performed with 7.1 mCi ^{99m}Tc-diphosphonate. The
images of the knees were obtained with the converging collimator and
were interpreted as being within normal limits, thus ruling out osteomyelitis. We have consistently seen negative bone scans in cases clinically believed to be traumatic or septic synovitis.

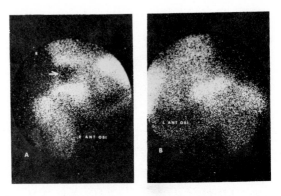

Fig. 10-12. Legg-Perthes disease. (A) Right anterior oblique view with pinhole collimator showing (arrow) avascular femoral head. (B) Normal left side.

Figure 10-12 shows the bone scan obtained in a 6-year-old boy who developed a painful right hip 5 weeks before this examination and who was clinically thought to have *Legg-Perthes disease.* The initial x-ray films were interpreted as being normal. At the time of the bone scan, the patient had flexor contraction of the right hip. The bone scan was performed with 7.2 mCi of ^{99m}Tc-diphosphonate to evaluate the vascularity of the femoral head. The absence of uptake in the right femoral head was seen in the anterior, anterior oblique, and posterior oblique projections. The images were for 100,000 counts and took less than 50 sec/image. The pinhole collimator images are superior in resolution to the converging collimator images. The avascular segment of the right femoral head is readily visualized in Fig. 10-12 which shows the anterior oblique views with the pinhole collimator. Our practice is to image the uninvolved side for 50,000 counts in the anterior projections and then to take all other images, anterior and anterior oblique images for both the uninvolved and involved sides for the same imaging time period. The patient was diagnosed as having Legg-Perthes disease and was treated appropriately by the orthopedic surgeons.

Summary

It was only a short time ago that bone scanning was restricted to only a relatively small number of nuclear medicine departments across the country. This reluctance on the part of the nuclear medicine physician to pursue bone scanning was due to the general unsatisfactory studies obtained with ^{85}Sr and ^{87m}Sr and to the cost and lack of universal availability of ^{18}F. The contribution of Subramanian represented a major breakthrough when ^{99m}Tc-polyphosphate was developed. This was shortly followed by other ^{99m}Tc-labeled phosphorous complexes: pyrophosphate, hydroxyethylidene disodium phosphonate, and methylene diphosphonate. At present all classes of ^{99m}Tc-labeled phosphorous complexes give comparable skeletal images, and the clinical experience gained from the use of any of the ^{99m}Tc-labeled compounds will aid in interpretation of the studies performed with the use of the others. However, there are differences in the ease and uniformity of preparation of the complexes and their respective blood clearance rates. In consideration of these differences, the agents of choice appear to be either hydroxyethylidene disodium phosphonate (9) or methylene diphosphonate (15). Now that the doors have been literally opened so that even the most modest nuclear medicine facilities may practice with "state of the art" radiopharmaceuticals, we will all gain from the necessarily large increase in available clinical studies. With the increase in clinical material, more rational determinations may be made of the role of bone scanning in the diagnosis and evaluation of efficacy of treatment in pediatric bone and joint diseases.

Examination of the modest number of clinical studies illustrated in this chapter will indicate the meager information that is known today. It should be clear to the reader that little is known and that there is much to be learned. The role of serial bone scanning in certain disease states, such as Legg-Calve-Perthes disease, will hopefully provide information on the mechanism of the disease as well as the role of treatment in interrupting the natural course of the disease.

It is reasonable to suggest that bone scanning provides information on the extent of primary bone tumors, on possible metastatic disease, on the presence of osteomyelitis prior to roentgenographic changes such that earlier therapy is possible, on the presence of collagen diseases, on the presence of fractures not disclosed by x-ray films, and on the evaluation of aseptic necrosis. However, the total effect and contribution of bone scanning to the diagnosis, treatment, and ultimate prognosis of pediatric skeletal diseases is, as yet, unknown. Hopefully some of these questions will be answered within the next few years.

References

1. McAfee JG, Subramanian G: Radioactive agents for the delineation of body organs by external imaging devices: a review. *ISA Transactions* 5: 349–372, 1966

2. Neuman WF, Neuman MW: The nature of the mineral phase of bone. *Chem Rev* 53: 1–45, 1953

3. Neuman WF, Neuman MW: *The Chemical Dynamics of Bone Mineral*. Chaps. 4 and 5. Chicago, University of Chicago Press, 1958

4. Van Dyke D, Anger HO, Yano Y, et al: Bone blood flow shown with fluorine-18 in the positron camera. *Am J Physiol* 209: 65–70, 1965

5. Blau M, Nagler W: Fluorine-18: a new isotope for bone scanning. *J Nucl Med* 3: 332–334, 1962

6. WHITLEY JE, WITCOFSKI RL, BOLLIGER TT, et al: Tc-99m in the visualization of neoplasms outside the brain. *Am J Roentgenol Radium Ther Nucl Med* 96: 706–710, 1966

7. SUBRAMANIAN G, MCAFEE JG, BELL EG, et al: Tc-99m labeled polyphosphate as a skeletal imaging agent. *Radiology* 102: 701–704, 1972

8. PEREZ R, COHEN Y, HENRY R, et al: A new radiopharmaceutical for ^{99m}Tc bone scanning. *J Nucl Med* 13: 788–789, 1972

9. CASTRONOVO FP, CALLAHAN RJ: New bone scanning agent: ^{99m}Tc-labeled 1-hydroxy-ethylidene-1,1-disodium phosphonate. *J Nucl Med* 13: 823–827, 1972

10. COMAR CL, LOTZ WE, BOYD GA: Autoradiographic studies on calcium, phosphorus and strontium distribution in the bones of the growing pig. *Am J Anat* 90: 113–129, 1952

11. BAUER GCH: The importance of bone growth as a factor in the redistribution of bone salt. *J Bone Joint Surg* 36A: 375–380, 1954

12. BELL EG, MCAFEE JG, SUBRAMANIAN G: Radiopharmaceuticals in pediatrics. In *Pediatric Nuclear Medicine.* James AE, Wagner HN, Cooke EC, eds, Philadelphia, WB Saunders, 1974

13. BUTLER AM, RITCHIE RH: Simplification and improvement in estimating drug dosage and fluid and dietary allowances for patients of varying sizes. *N Engl J Med* 262: 903–908, 1960

14. BELL EG, MCAFEE JG, CONSTABLE WC: Local radiation damage to bone and marrow demonstrated by radioisotopic imaging. *Radiology,* 92: 1083–1088, 1969

15. SUBBRAMANIAN G, BLAIR RJ, KALLFELZ EJ, et al: ^{99m}Tc methylene diphosphonate (MDP): A superior agent for skeletal imaging. *J Nucl Med* 14: 640, 1973

Chapter **11**

Tumor

Eugene T. Morita

The tumor (T), node (N), and distant metastases (M) classification was developed to provide a more objective means for staging various tumors. It provides a standard procedure for comparing various tumors in different institutions. The efficacy of treatment plans and prognosis can be better evaluated by uniform staging procedures.

Nuclear medicine offers clinicians a means by which the primary tumor, nodes, and distant metastases can be evaluated. The primary tumor is occasionally evaluated but the use is somewhat hampered by limitations of resolution. Thyroid nodules are frequently evaluated, however, because of the importance of their function with respect to their uptake of radioiodine (nonfunctioning nodules have a higher incidence of tumor). In children, nodules are more suspect for tumor since there is a higher incidence of tumors in nodules in childhood. The child with a thyroid nodule and a history of previous ionizing radiation to the head or neck has a higher incidence of thyroid carcinoma. Nuclear medicine procedures offer a relatively noninvasive means of evaluating the primary tumor.

Nodal involvement (N) can be evaluated with radionuclide procedures, but these have not achieved widespread use or acceptance. Colloidal ^{198}Au and other radioactive colloids have been used to identify intra-abdominal nodes but these have been of limited usefulness. Radioiodine has been exceedingly useful in defining metastatic thyroid carcinoma in the neck and mediastinum in patients with functioning thyroid carcinoma. Adequate levels of thyroid stimulating hormone are required. Gallium-citrate has been used by some clinics to define Hodgkin's involvement in the mediastinum and abdomen (1). We are frequently called upon to evaluate distant metastases (M) with the use of various large organ imaging techniques. The brain, bone, and liver imaging studies have been widely used in determining the presence and extent of distant metastases. It seems reasonable that if primary tumors are associated with distant metastases, different therapeutic approaches might be undertaken.

Thyroid Carcinoma

Since the development of ^{131}I in the diagnosis and treatment of functioning thyroid carcinoma, no other tumor specific agents have been found. Thyroid carcinoma in childhood usually presents as a nodule in the thyroid gland and in some series 80% show evidence of regional metastases, with 20% of the patients having evidence of pulmonary metastases on routine chest x-ray at the time of initial evaluation (2). Because most differentiated thyroid carcinomas of childhood do not function with respect to their uptake of ^{131}I, surgical removal of normal thyroid tissue or radioablation is necessary to induce function in metastatic foci (3). The rationale for recommending total thyroidectomy in patients with thyroid carcinoma are for the following reasons: (A) total thyroidectomy removes virtually all normal thyroid tissue and bulk tumor which might compete for radioiodine in diagnostic and therapeutic modalities, (B) removal of all normally functioning tissue decreases the whole-body radiation dose given to the patient since less protein-bound ^{131}I enters the systemic circulation, and (C) tumors in the contralateral lobe have been reported in some patients (3, 4). After the removal of thyroid tissue, high levels of endogenous TSH often induce uptake of radioactive iodine in metastatic foci (2, 3). Functioning metastatic carcinoma to the lungs following the oral ingestion of ^{131}I has been reported in the face of a negative chest x-ray (5). In some reports it has been described as being unusual. Recent studies have shown that these findings represent an early stage of metastatic disease to the lungs. The most common presentation of a differentiated thyroid carcinoma, metastatic to the lungs, is that of a diffuse miliary pattern (6). Recently three patients from Letterman General Hospital and the University of California Medical Center were found to have this pattern. One patient underwent lung biopsy and was found to have multiple small metastatic foci in the lungs with associated positive autoradiographs (7). The finding of a positive ^{131}I scan in the face of a negative chest x-ray represents an early stage of metastatic carcinoma to the lungs (Fig. 11-1). The work by Varma, et al (8) suggests that those patients over the age of 40 who respond to ^{131}I do considerably better than those who do not. Differentiated thyroid carcinoma becomes progressively more aggressive when initially diagnosed in the older age group. It therefore seems reasonable that therapy with ^{131}I in

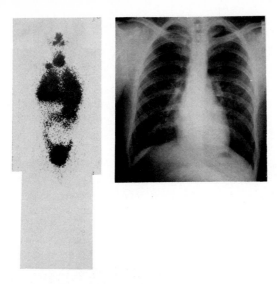

Fig. 11-1. (Left) Whole-body scan (anterior). (Right) Radiograph (PA) of young man with differentiated carcinoma of thyroid, proven at lung biopsy to have metastatic lung implants. Radioiodine scan (left) shows diffuse activity in right supraclavicular node and lungs. Chest films (right) were normal.

those patients with functioning thyroid carcinoma gives a greater likelihood of survival.

Tumor Localization

Tumor abnormalities on large organ images are seen because of anatomic alterations and/or altered physiology. Alteration of the physiology may be due to the changes caused by the tumor or by active uptake by the tumor itself. The anatomic defects seen in large organ imaging will be covered in other chapters, but there are a few findings which may be of interest in this section. The finding of a "hot spot" on the liver scan in patients with mediastinal masses has been recently reported in the literature. This "hot spot" is due to high-specific-activity radiopharmaceutical entering the venous collaterals and entering the terminal branches of the portal circulation in the region of the porta hepatis (9, 10). A second finding which is occasionally seen in patients with malignant disease is that of hepatic vein thrombosis.

Anatomically, the venous drainage from the caudate lobe of the liver, unlike the other lobes, enters the vena cava directly rather than through the hepatic vein (11). The caudate lobe is thus spared the congestion which the other lobes suffer. The finding on the scan is that of prominence of the midportion of the liver near the midline corresponding to the caudate lobe. There are presently insufficient cases in the litera-

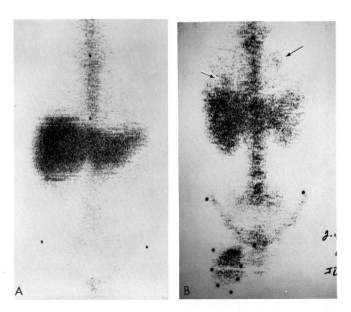

Fig. 11-2. (A) Normal anterior view whole-body scan after injection of ^{111}In-bleomycin. Note normal accumulation in liver, sternum, and pelvic marrow. (B) Whole-body scan 48 hr postinjection with ^{111}In-bleomycin. 19-year-old man with rhabdomyosarcoma of anterior right thigh. Note primary lesion surrounded by black dots in anterior right thigh, but more important, right lower lobe and left upper lobe accumulations indicative of metastatic disease (arrows). (Courtesy of L. R. Bennett, UCLA.)

ture to appreciate the changes which might occur in these patients with time.

Under defects noted because of physiological alterations, the subject will be limited to those in which there is active uptake of the radionuclide by tumor. As previously mentioned, ^{131}I is the only *specific* agent which is presently used for the diagnosis of tumor. Nonspecific agents which might be used in the staging of childhood tumors are ^{75}Se-selenomethionine, ^{67}Ga-citrate, ^{111}In-chloride, and recently, bleomycin labeled with ^{99m}Tc or [111]In.

Selenium-75 has been used by Cavalieri for the definition of malignant tumors (*12*). Selenomethionine has been used by some investigators in defining nonfunctioning thyroid nodules (*13*). Certain tumors in many of the patients revealed function with respect to uptake of selenomethionine as compared to the nonfunctioning ^{131}I scan. Recent studies with ^{67}Ga-citrate suggest that metastatic foci may be delineated with the use of this radionuclide.

Gallium-67-citrate has been frequently used in the staging of various lymphomas. The mechanism of action is thought to be related to transfer into cells of high lysosomal activity and is partly a function of blood flow to the area (*14, 15*). The radionuclide appears to be nonspecific in nature in that it is taken up by a myriad of tumors, both meta-static and primary. Abscesses have been found with the use of ^{67}Ga-citrate and are thought to be a function of the leukocyte metabolism.

Indium-111-chloride labels to transferrin when given intravenously, and some preliminary work done by Goodwin suggests that it may be useful as a tumor imaging agent in that it localizes in certain tumors (16).

Bleomycin, a new tumor antibiotic, has been useful in the treatment of various adult tumors such as carcinoma of the lung, squamous cell tumors, and lymphomas. Bleomycin has been labeled with ^{99m}Tc and ^{111}In, and much preliminary work is occurring at the present time (17, 18) (Fig. 11-2). It remains to be seen whether labeled bleomycin will be effective in localizing specific pediatric tumors.

Ray and his coworkers have reported a case of aspergillus niger in-fection which was detected by the use of [85]Sr (19). Subsequent tissue studies of the organism revealed high concentration in the areas noted on scan. A similar unpublished case was noted at Fitzsimmons General Hospital in a patient with a bronchogenic carcinoma with an associated aspergillus flavus infection. Strontium-87m has been shown by Samuels to be taken up by osteogenic tumors metastatic to the lungs (20). A re-cent case from Letterman General Hospital revealed a similar patient with metastatic pulmonary disease from an osteogenic sarcoma (21). The radiopharmaceutical used in this patient was ^{99m}Tc-polyphosphate. The use of bone seeking agents may be useful in following patients with such tumors in associated metastasis before they are roentgenographically noted. A problem, however, is that differentiation between pulmonary uptake and rib uptake must be made. The bone scan for evaluation of bony involvement is of proven usefulness in patients with metastatic disease.

In addition to a particular radionuclide used for a diagnosis, com-bined studies either in the form of temporal sequence or different com-binations of radionuclides have proven useful. Temporal relationships have been used in nuclear medicine, particularly in brain imaging. Handa has found that the tumor-to-background ratio is different in tumors of a vascular variety than in patients with less vascular tumors and strokes (22). Conway has defined pediatric mediastinal lesions by the use of sequential studies and has found them very useful in defining whether they are cystic, solid, or vascular (23). Cystic lesions are negative through-out the time sequence study whereas vascular tumors function through-out the sequence. The series is small but the technique appears to be very useful.

Combined radionuclide studies, such as ^{99m}Tc-sulfur colloid liver scans used in conjunction with ^{67}Ga-citrate, may be of value. Hepatomas and other metastatic tumors to the liver show defects on colloid scanning whereas the ^{67}Ga-citrate study reveals uptake by the tumor (15). Shoop has found a functioning hepatoma with rose bengal which revealed a negative defect with the colloid scan (24).

High-Risk Patient

In addition to the actual staging procedure in childhood tumors and the search for metastases at a later date, radionuclide studies are useful in patients who are predisposed to certain tumors. Identical twins with tumors such as leukemias have been noted in the literature. In children with Bloom syndrome, Downs syndrome, and survivors within one thousand meters of the Hiroshima atomic bomb blast, there is an increased incidence of leukemia. In patients with congenital hemihypertrophy it is known that Wilms' tumors, primary hepatic tumors, and adrenal cortical neoplasia occur with increased frequency (25). Patients with tuberous sclerosis and multiple neurofibromatosis have been found to develop brain tumors. Young children with basal cell nevus syndrome and their related but unaffected siblings have developed medulloblastomas. Patients with Wiscott-Aldrich syndrome and ataxia telangiectasia have been found to have astrocytomas and medulloblastomas, respectively. Familial medullary carcinoma of the thyroid has been known to occur and microscopic tumors of medullary variety have been found in those with no physical findings. As the list of patients with both familial and environmental factors which would predispose to malignancy grows, greater use of radioisotope studies may help detect the diseases at an earlier stage.

Much has been accomplished in pediatric nuclear medicine with respect to the imaging of various tumors of childhood, but aside from ^{131}I no other tumor specific agents have been found. It is apparent both intuitively and from a biological standpoint that tumors which specifically take up radionuclides are more readily detected than those that leave a void as a manifestation of the tumor. Although the present limitations of our equipment at best is 1 cm, lesions smaller than this size can be detected if the tumor uptake of the radionuclide is sufficiently greater than that of background. Hence, it seems imminently reasonable that a greater search for such agents be undertaken.

Summary

Imaging procedures offer a relatively noninvasive means by which a primary tumor and evidence of nodal or distant metastasis can be assessed. Nodal involvement is difficult to assess except for those which take up material actively such as ^{131}I in thyroid carcinoma and ^{67}Ga-citrate in lymphomas. Those patients in whom tumors have a familial relationship or predisposition can be evaluated. Significant breakthroughs in detection of tumors will occur with the development of additional tumor specific agents.

References

1. TURNER DA, PINSKY SM, GOTTSHALK A, et al: The use of gallium-67 scanning in the staging of Hodgkin's disease. *Radiology* 103: 97–100, 1972

2. EXELBY PE, FRAZELL EL: Carcinoma of the thyroid in children. *Surg Clin North Am* 49: 249–259, 1969

3. POCHIN EE: Prospects from the treatment of thyroid carcinoma with radioiodine. *Clin Radiol* 18: 113–135, 1967

4. RUSSELL WO, IBANE ML, CLARK RL, et al: Thyroid carcinoma, classification, intraglandular dissemination and clinicopathological study based upon whole organ section of eighty glands. *Cancer* 160: 1425–1460, 1963

5. BARRETT O, STENBERG ES: Pulmonary metastases from thyroid carcinoma: an unusual case. *Ann Intern Med* 62: 767–770, 1965

6. MacDONALD JS: X-ray diagnosis. In *Tumors of the Thyroid Gland,* vol 6, Smithers D, ed, Edinburgh & London, Livingston E S, 1970, pp 189–201

7. MORITA ET: Unpublished data, 1973

8. VARMA VM, BEIERWALTES WH, NOFAL MM: Treatment of thyroid cancer. *JAMA* 214: 1437–1442, 1970

9. MORITA ET, McCORMACK KR, WEISBERG RL: Further information on the "hot spot" in the liver. *J Nucl Med* 14: 606–608, 1973

10. JOYNER J: Abnormal liver scan (radiocolloid "hot spot") associated with superior vena caval obstruction. *J Nucl Med* 13: 849–851, 1972

11. JONES EJ: Hepatic scintillography. *Gut* 8: 418–420, 1967

12. CAVALIERI R, SCOTT KG: Sodium selenite Se-75. *JAMA* 106: 591–595, 1968

13. THOMAS CG, PEPPER FD, OWEN J, et al: Differentiation of malignancy from benign lesions of the thyroid gland using complementary scanning with selenomethionine 75 and radioiodine. *Ann Surg* 170: 396–408, 1969

14. SWARTZENDRUBER DC, NELSON B, HAYES RL, et al: Gallium-67 localization in lysomal-like granules of leukemia and nonleukemic murine tissues. *JNCI* 46: 941–947, 1971

15. SUZUKI T, HNOJO I, et al: Positive scintiphotography of cancer of the liver with gallium-67 citrate. *Am J Roentgenol Radium Ther Nucl Med* 113: 92–103, 1971

16. GOODWIN D, GOODE R, BROWN L, et al: Indium 111-labeled transferrin for the detection of tumor. *Radiology* 100: 157–179, 1971

17. BUSSE J. ^{99m}Tc-bleomycin tumor imaging. Paper presented Stanford Nuclear Medicine Conference, December 20, 1972

18. RENAULT H, RAPIN J, RUDLER M, et al: Labeling method using the chelation of various radioactive cations by some polypeptides: Application to bleomycin. *Chim Ther* 7: 232–235, 1972

19. RAY GR, DeNARDO GL, KING GH: Localization of Sr 85 in soft tissues infected by Aspergillus niger. *Radiology* 101: 119–123, 1971

20. SAMUELS LD: Lung scanning with Sr-87m in metastatic osteosarcoma. *Am J Roentgenol Radium Ther Nucl Med* 104: 766–769, 1968

21. LAWSON M: Personal communication. 1973

22. HANDA J, NABESHIMA S, HANDA H, et al: Serial brain scanning with Tc^{99m} and the scintillation camera. *Am J Roentgenol Radium Ther Nucl Med* 106: 708–723, 1969

23. CONWAY JJ, SHERMAN JO: Evaluation of chest masses in children with early and delayed radionuclide angiography. *Am J Roentgenol Radium Ther Nucl Med* 108: 575–581, 1970

24. SHOOP J: Functional hepatoma demonstrated with rose bengal. *Am J Roentgenol Radium Ther Nucl Med* 107: 51–53, 1969

25. MILLER RW: Epidemiology of childhood neoplasia. In *Neoplasia in Childhood,* 12th Annual Clinical Conf. Chicago, Ill. Yearbook Publishers, 1969, pp 13–24

Discussion

Daniel B. Schere (Children's Hospital, Buenos Aires, Argentina): Do you have any experience (or does anyone) in detecting neuroblastoma with specific radionuclides?

Dr. Morita: I don't. [Editor's note: Samuels alludes to a case where the mediastinal widening seen on [87m]Sr scanning was later found to be a neuroblastoma (Samuels CD: Detection and localization of extra skeletal malignant neoplasms of children with strontium-87m. *Am J Roentgenol Radium Ther Nucl Med* 115: 777–782, 1972.) Conventional radiography has done so well that we are usually not asked to evaluate these children. Robert O'Mara at the Arizona Medical Center has imaged neuroblastomas in children with both [67]Ga- and ^{111}In-bleomycin (personal communication).

Uptake has been noted in a patient with a neuroblastoma having a ^{99m}Tc bone scan. The surgical specimen of the tumor showed calcification on histologic examination.]

Chapter 12

Hematology

David C. Price and Curt Ries

The performance of standard radioisotopic hematologic procedures in the evaluation of pediatric disease states does not differ fundamentally from their performance in adult populations. Two factors, however, do introduce modifications which must be considered: radiation exposure is a much more sensitive factor in children, and the spectrum of hematologic diseases to be evaluated is distinctly different from that in adults. This review is designed to outline the radioisotopic hematologic techniques in current use, to detail our own clinical experience with these techniques over the past several years, and to indicate some newer methods which are just now being applied to pediatric investigation and which would appear to have an important future in this field.

Radiation Dosimetry

Table 12-1 summarizes the various radiopharmaceuticals in current use in pediatric hematologic diagnosis, giving the amount of radioisotope administered in μCi/kg and the associated whole-body radiation dose at ages ranging from newborn to adulthood. These figures have been derived almost entirely from Refs. 1–5 which also in some instances detail critical organ dosimetry. Blanks have been left where radiation dose calculations were not available, and in the case of ^{99m}Tc-sulfur colloid the figures in parentheses represent calculations extrapolated from dosimetry in the adult, assuming similar organ distributions and diminishing total-body size in younger age groups. The dosimetry stated is based upon varying

TABLE 12-1. Whole-Body Radiation Dose from Hematologic Radiopharmaceuticals (milliroentgens)*

Radiopharmaceutical	Dose (μCi/kg)	Newborn	1 Year	5 Years	10 Years	15 Years	Adult
^{51}Cr-RBC (red cell surv.)	1.43	35	43	44	48	47	50
^{99m}Tc-RBC	4.29	3.0	3.6	3.5	4.3	4.7	6.0
^{125}I-IHSA	0.071	6.6	7.2	7.3	7.6	7.8	8.0
^{131}I-IHSA	0.071	8.1	8.6	8.7	9.6	9.4	10.0
^{99m}Tc-albumin	4.29	3.0	3.6	3.5	4.3	4.7	6.0
^{113m}In-transferrin	14.3						16
^{59}Fe (oral)	0.14	20	26	26	28	31	34
^{59}Fe (i.v.)	0.14	147	190	189	201	212	230
^{55}Fe (i.v.)	0.14						(410)
^{57}Co-B$_{12}$	0.007	1.4	1.9	2.0	2.2	2.4	2.7
^{60}Co-B$_{12}$	0.007	61	86	91	98	106	120
^{99m}Tc-sulfur-colloid	85.7	(51)	(70)	(75)	(82)	(90)	100
IVP		90	190	310	480	890	970
UGI, BE		300	480	720	1100	1300	1400

* Data from Refs. 1 to 5.

the amount of radioisotope by body weight, but more constant dosimetry at different ages would result if the administered amount of tracer were to be calculated by surface area. Although there is no absolute upper limit of safety for radiation dosimetry in pediatrics, it is quite evident that some tracers are associated with a much lower radiation dose than others, a factor which must be considered in undertaking radioisotopic studies in children.

Blood Volume Procedure

The blood volume in man is a heterogeneous compartment, most readily subdivided for tracer evaluation into plasma volume and red cell mass. Each of these spaces can and should be evaluated by the dilutional assay principle, using a protein tag for plasma volume and a red cell tracer for red cell mass. Because of variations in the hematocrit in different body organs, the ratio of whole-body hematocrit to venous hematocrit is not unity. This ratio is defined as the F_{cell} ratio and has been calculated to vary widely from 0.720 to 1.005 (± 2 s.d.), the median being in the range of 0.860 (6)–0.915 (7). Thus it is possible in a given patient to introduce an error as large as 5–20% in blood volume estimation by measuring only one of the two intravascular spaces. Also, as has been emphasized by others, the venous hematocrit determination itself must be corrected for plasma trapping in the red cell column, a correction factor of 0.96 generally being used.

The most widely used tracer for plasma volume determination is ^{125}I-radioiodinated human serum albumin (IHSA), 0.07 μCi/kg body weight. This has largely replaced ^{131}I-IHSA, which has a shorter half-life and greater patient irradiation. The tracer is injected intravenously with the patient in the resting state and supine, and the dilutional volume is calculated from a plasma sample taken 10 min after injection. Although this is adequate time for complete plasma mixing, an additional correction may have to be made if considerable albumin loss is occurring through the gastrointestinal or genitourinary tracts. Plasma volume may also be calculated with higher counting rates and consequently better statistical accuracy using ^{99m}Tc-albumin, 4.3 μCi/kg, or [113m]In-transferrin, 14.3 μCi/kg. In the latter case, the indium may be bound to the patient's own transferrin if it is not fully saturated with iron, or even administered directly intravenously if there are adequate transferrin binding sites available.

Red cell mass must be estimated by labeling the patient's own red blood cells under sterile conditions with ^{51}Cr as sodium chromate, 0.43 μCi/kg, or more recently ^{99m}Tc as pertechnetate (usually in the presence of stannous chloride), 4.3 μCi/kg (8). Autologous blood is drawn into ACD solution B under sterile conditions, and the radiotracer is added in appropriate dose and incubated at room temperature for 30–45 min. Ascorbic acid, 100 mg, can be introduced at the end of this time to reduce all unbound hexavalent chromium although this step is not necessary with red cell washing. The tagged red cells are then washed three times with normal saline, and a measured aliquot is re-injected into the patient in the resting state with retention of a standard for calculation. Although complete mixing generally occurs within 15 min, certain disease states, particularly the presence of splenomegaly, will delay this mixing and make it advisable to use a 40-min sample for the dilutional assay.

The following equations are used in calculations of the blood volume:

$$\text{Plasma volume} = \frac{(\text{Total cpm } ^{125}\text{I-IHSA injected})}{(\text{cpm } ^{125}\text{I-IHSA/cc plasma at 10 min})}$$

$$\text{Red cell mass} = \frac{(\text{Total cpm } ^{51}\text{Cr-RBC injected}) \times (\text{HCT}) \times (0.96)}{(\text{cpm } ^{51}\text{Cr-RBC/cc whole blood at 40 min})}$$

Blood volume

$$= \text{Red cell mass } (^{51}\text{Cr}) + \text{Plasma volume } (^{125}\text{I-IHSA}).$$

When only the plasma volume has been specifically measured:

$$\text{Blood volume} = \frac{\text{Plasma volume}}{1 - (\text{HCT}) \times (0.96) \times (0.915)}.$$

When only the red cell mass has been measured:

$$\text{Blood volume} = \frac{\text{Red cell mass}}{(\text{HCT}) \times (0.96) \times (0.915)}.$$

In the last two equations, 0.915 has been used as the F_{cell} ratio, and the hematocrits are expressed as a fraction rather than a percent.

Although one of the early, commonly used radioisotopic techniques in hematology, the blood-volume determination by both of these methods appears now to be less and less frequently requested. Our laboratory has performed 159 blood volumes over the past 4 years, an average of 40 per year, of which 87% were ^{125}I-IHSA plasma volumes, and 13% were ^{51}Cr red cell mass determinations. Whereas in the past the common reason for determining blood volume was pre- and postsurgical assessment, of these 159 determinations 41% were in children with renal transplants, and 15% were in children with hypertension. The evaluation of polycythemia, one of the most important reasons for blood volume measurement in adults, is a rare occurrence in the pediatric population.

Red Blood Cell Survival Studies

Although not a true tracer of the red cell throughout its life span, the most practical radioisotope for red cell survival studies is nevertheless ^{51}Cr in the form of sodium chromate. When incubated with autologous red blood cells in ACD under sterile conditions as described for determination of the red cell mass, 80–90% of the radiochromium diffuses across the red cell membrane, is reduced inside the cell, and binds mainly to the beta chain of globin. The determination of red cell survival is begun the day following injection of the labeled cells since 2–10% of the tracer will elute from the red cells in the first 24 hr. There is an additional, relatively constant elution rate of approximately 1% (0.6–2.3%) per day from the labeled red cells (9) as well as the 0.83% per day loss by cell death. As a result, the time to reach 50% of the 24-hr blood activity level is not 60 days as one would expect with the 120-day lifespan of red cells, but approximately 30 days (range 25–35 days).

External counting is an extremely important component of the red cell survival study in evaluating the role of the spleen in hemolytic states. Of great importance in external counting is the fact that the normal spleen is a posterior organ and should be counted posteriorly or laterally unless it is substantially enlarged and palpable anteriorly. The most effective technique for deciding external counting sites is to inject a small amount of ^{99m}Tc-sulfur colloid 24 hr before the chromium study, and scan the liver-spleen area anteriorly and posteriorly, thus defining the optimum counting locations over the liver and spleen. A larger amount of ^{51}Cr is used than in the red cell mass determination, 1.4 μCi/kg, since the study may extend over several weeks. As mentioned previously, except for blood samples at 10 and 40 min to determine red cell mass, the red cell survival counting is not begun until 24 hr after tracer injection. Blood samples are obtained at 24, 48, and 72 hr and counted to see if an extremely rapid disappearance half-time is present. Subsequent sampling times are determined by this initial rate of disappearance, generally three times a week for 3 weeks. Counts over spleen and liver are performed with a 3 × 2-in. NaI(Tl) crystal and flat field collimator, at 24 hr, 72 hr, and once or twice weekly thereafter until approximately one half-life has been reached. Most important in evaluating splenic sequestration is the observation of a rising spleen: liver ratio throughout the study, rather than any single high ratio.

Table 12-2 summarizes our own experience with red cell survival studies in seven children over the past 4 years, including a 20-year-old man with Gilbert's disease having a red cell half-time of 29.8 days to represent the normal. Of the two patients who were studied before and after splenectomy, it is interesting to note that the child with thalassemia major (JC) had a high spleen-to-liver ratio which did not rise throughout the time of study, and she demonstrated very little increase in red cell half-time following splenectomy. On the other hand, the child with hereditary spherocytosis (DL) essentially doubled the spleen-to-liver ratio before splenectomy, and continuation of counts over the week following splenectomy indicated a major improvement in red cell life span. The figure of 39.7 days is unusually high because only four data points could be obtained in the four immediate postoperative days.

Figure 12-1 summarizes the counting data in Patient JC before and after splenectomy, and illustrates one extremely important factor essential to the evaluation of red cell survival half-time. It is optimal, some people believe essential, for the patient to be in a stable hematologic state during the time of study. If this is so, then minor daily fluctuations in hematocrit can be smoothed by dividing each blood count by the hematocrit on that date, generally giving a much closer fit to a straight line on semilogarithmic plot. If, however, as in Patient JC, the hematocrit is falling during the time of study, correcting the individual day's ^{51}Cr count by its hematocrit will erroneously lengthen the half-time. In this case a more valid index of survival half-time will be obtained from whole-blood activity in spite of the falling hematocrit. Thus in Fig. 12-1, the half-time before splenectomy was 7.1 days using whole-blood samples, but virtually within normal limits (24 days) if corrected for hematocrit variations. To reiterate, whole blood ^{51}Cr counts should be corrected for hematocrit variations in the steady state but should not be corrected for hematocrit variations if there is a steadily rising or falling hematocrit.

Other methods of cell labeling are available for red cell survival studies, but none of these permits external counting to evaluate splenic sequestration. DF ^{32}P (the cholinesterase inhibitor diisopropylfluorophosphate-^{32}P) binds in vitro or less preferably in vivo to cholinesterase in the

TABLE 12-2. Red Blood Cell Survival Studies in Children

Patient	Age	Red cell half-time (days)	Spleen/liver ratio	Diagnosis
FM	20 yr	29.8		Gilbert's disease
RB	17 yr	9.4		Nonspherocytic hemolytic anemia
JC	6 yr	7.1	8–8	Thalassemia major
		12	0	Postsplenectomy
ME	6 mo	5.4	1.8–2.2	Osteopetrosis, pancytopenia
JJ	16 mo	4.1	0	Thalassemia major, spleen out
DL	2 yr	8.0	1.5–2.9	Hereditary spherocytosis
		39.7	0	Postsplenectomy
JM	2 yr	3.7	0.5–2.1	Hemolytic anemia
KM	15 yr	6.9	1.0–1.2	Coombs positive hemolytic anemia
		13.7		Retics dropping

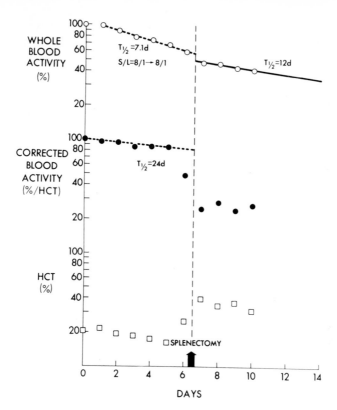

Fig. 12-1. ^{51}Cr-tagged red blood survival study in JC, 6-year-old child with thalassemia major, before and after splenectomy. Absence of significant rise in spleen-to-liver ratio is associated with little change in red cell survival half-time following surgery.

red cell membrane and has almost no elution rate, so that a more physiologic value for the red cell survival half-time can be obtained. This radiopharmaceutical is highly toxic, however, in anything other than tiny doses. Other red cell labels including glycine-2-^{14}C, ^{75}Se-selenomethionine, etc., have been used investigatively but cannot be considered to be routine diagnostic tracers.

Platelet Survival Studies

Platelet labeling can be performed in the same manner as the labeling of red cells although the high binding capability of chromium to red cells requires initial separation of the platelets by differential centrifugation (*10, 11*). Chromium-51 as sodium chromate, 4.3 μCi/kg, is added to the platelet-rich plasma separated from 100 to 450 ml of blood. This is followed by incubation for 1 hr at room temperature, washing of the platelets three times, and reinfusion of the tagged platelets suspended in plasma. Unlike the red cell tagging procedure, only 10–30% of the tracer ultimately binds to platelets and is returned to the patient. It is preferable to use autologous platelets because of the much greater complexity of platelet typing and the possibility of platelet isoantibodies in patients with thrombocytopenia and previous transfusions. When the platelet count is particularly low (less than 20,000–30,000), donor platelets may have to be used, in which case HL-A typing and matching is an important adjunct to the study.

Since the normal platelet life span is slightly under 10 days and since many patients being evaluated will have half-lives of hours rather than days, the blood sampling and external counting performed in a platelet kinetic study are similar in format to a red cell survival study but considerably condensed in time. Where accelerated platelet destruction is anticipated, blood samples are drawn 10, 20, 30, 60, 90, 120, 180, and 240 min after injection of the labeled platelets, with external spleen and liver counting performed at several points along this time schedule. An additional blood sample and external count are performed at 24 hr, then if still indicated at 48, 72, 96, and 120 hr, or to one half-time.

As with the red cell survival study, the significance of external counting lies in a rising spleen-to-liver ratio rather than any single high ratio. Once again, posterior or lateral spleen counting is essential in the absence of splenomegaly. Two features of the blood disappearance data are important. First, there is usually a rapid fall in blood platelet specific activity in the first 15 min with a slower half-time thereafter, back-extrapolation of this final slope being used to calculate the total amount of injected labeled platelets accountable for in blood at equilibration. This figure, compared with the total injected platelet radioactivity and expressed as the percent platelet recovery, normally averages 70% of total platelets injected. The value approaches 100% in the absence of the spleen and falls much lower than 70% in the presence of splenomegaly. Second, the

TABLE 12-3. Platelet Kinetics in Children

Patient	Age	Platelet $T_{1/2}$	% recovery	Spleen/liver	Diagnosis
MB	5 mo	5.3 hr	37	±	Hepatosplenomegaly, AML
DC	5 yr	32 hr	77	++	ITP
MH	9½ yr	2.2 d	32	+	Renal transplant
MK	17 mo	4.0 hr	94	(Splx)	Hem. anemia? DIC
TM	6 yr	2.7 hr	59	+++	Chronic ITP; Plat 6,000
	6½ yr	2.3 d	100	(Splx)	Plat 200,000

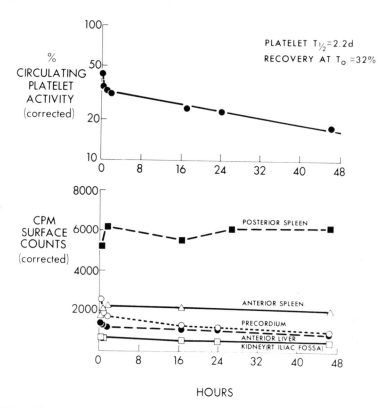

Fig. 12-2. ^{51}Cr-tagged platelet survival study in MH, 9-year-old renal transplant patient with recent thrombocytopenia. There is slight splenic pooling (recovery 32%) and slight shortening of survival half-time (2.2 days) but no evidence of progressive platelet sequestration in either spleen or transplant.

disappearance of blood activity after 15–30 min, although more linear than logarithmic in normals, is customarily expressed as the survival half-time as in red cell survival studies, the normal half-time averaging 96 hr. Finally, from the half-time a rate constant can be calculated, and from blood platelet count and plasma volume estimation the rate of platelet production per day can be estimated.

Table 12-3 summarizes the platelet kinetic studies performed in five children to date in our laboratory. As noted in Patients DC and TM, ITP is customarily associated with a markedly shortened platelet half-time, positive splenic sequestration by external counting, and marked improvement following splenectomy. As seen in Patient MH, the presence of splenomegaly alone is characteristically associated with a low percent recovery and a normal or almost normal survival half-time, splenic pooling resulting in a low circulating platelet count. Diseases such as DIC, suspected in Patient MK, result in rapid platelet disappearance presumably due to peripheral utilization. Thus, although the procedure is complex to undertake, it gives important information in thrombocytopenic states as to whether the primary defect is in production or utilization, and whether the spleen appears to play a role in platelet pooling or destruction.

Figure 12-2 illustrates the plasma platelet radioactivity in Patient MH, demonstrating rapid equilibration with the large splenic pool and a consequent platelet recovery of 32%, then a survival half-time of 2.2 days which is only slightly shorter than normal. The external counting demonstrates rapid initial pooling in the spleen and no significant late splenic rise. In the external counting, note the much higher activity found over the spleen posteriorly, the progressive fall in precordial and liver activity, and the absence of significant activity over the transplanted kidney where it was suspected some platelet sequestration might be taking place. In Patient MK (Fig. 12-3) a markedly abbreviated half-time was noted. As a result of previous splenectomy, the platelet recovery was nearly 100%. With a concomitant hemolytic anemia, there was concern

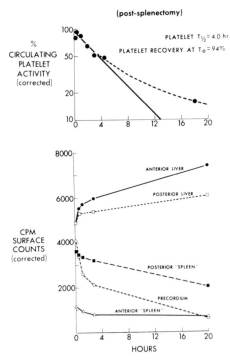

Fig. 12-3. ^{51}Cr-tagged platelet survival study in MK, splenectomized 17-month-old child with hemolytic anemia and suspected DIC or occult hemangioma. Note evidence of hepatic sequestration over 20 hr of study.

that this child might have an undiscovered large hemangioma with platelet sequestration and red cell destruction occurring in its vascular bed. Disseminated intravascular coagulation was the second major consideration. As illustrated in Fig. 12-4, using a Searle Radiographics Pho/Dot scanner with the central 19-hole cone removed from the collimator, it was possible to obtain quite an adequate whole-body scan demonstrating that the only definable site of platelet localization was the liver.

Leukocyte Survival Studies

It is possible to label both polymorphonuclear leukocytes and lymphocytes with ^{51}Cr as sodium chromate, or with DF-^{32}P (*12–14*). We have performed none of these studies to date in our laboratory, and so the techniques will not be reviewed here. As with platelet labeling, the main problem lies with the necessity to separate the specific cell types before labeling. This is a more complex problem with leukocytes where a variety of methods such as glass wool columns, metal filings, etc., are needed to separate the lymphocytes from the polymorphonuclear leukocytes after differential centrifugation has removed the red cells and platelets.

Fig. 12-4. Whole-body rectilinear scan of ^{51}Cr-tagged platelet distribution at 20 hr in patient MK (see Fig. 12-3). Note dominant hepatic localization and absence of any other focus of activity which might have suggested large hemangioma.

Ferrokinetics

Ferrokinetic studies in children are performed in the identical manner to adults. Iron-59 as ferrous citrate is the isotope of choice, at a dose of 0.14 μCi/kg. Iron-55 can be used for plasma radioiron disappearance and red cell incorporation, but its lack of gamma-ray emission obviates external counting for organ kinetics. Iron-52 is a positron emitter with a short half-life (8 hr) which is expensive and difficult to produce, requiring the availability of a cyclotron. Because of its half-life, it cannot be used beyond 24–36 hr in a kinetic study.

Because of the high gamma energies of ^{59}Fe and the small amounts of tracer used, a large sodium iodide crystal with heavy lead shielding gives maximum sensitivity and minimum nontarget background for external counting. We currently use the scanning head of a Searle Radiographics Pho/Dot scanner, which has a 3 × 2-in. NaI(Tl) crystal and lead shielding averaging 1½ in. in thickness around it. For collimation, removing the multihole insert from a 19-hole or 37-hole focusing collimator provides a tapered aperture 3¾ in. in diameter at the detector surface and 2 in. in diameter at the outside surface. Although this geometry does not give a highly localized region of sensitivity for external counting, it is seldom that high spatial resolution is necessary in a ferrokinetic study, and the increased sensitivity is extremely useful with the small radioiron doses used in children. To date we have performed two ferrokinetic studies in children and have found patterns over liver, spleen, and bone marrow sites which appear quite adequate in localization and information content for clinical evaluation.

As in the adult, the ferrokinetic study is begun by incubating the radioiron for 45 min with autologous plasma, then injecting a measured aliquot intravenously while retaining a portion for the standard. If the patient's transferrin is fully saturated, normal plasma from a nonhepatitic donor should be used. Prior scanning of the liver and spleen with ^{99m}Tc-sulfur colloid is again useful in localizing the counting points for these organs.

There are three major components to the ferrokinetic study:

1. The plasma radioiron disappearance curve is determined by counting 0.5–1.0-cc plasma samples drawn at 10, 20, 30, 60, 120, and 240 min after tracer injection. The daily plasma iron turnover (PIT) may then be calculated using the plasma volume (PV) measured with ^{125}I-IHSA or Evans blue dye, and the serum iron (SI) as follows:

$$\text{PIT (mg/day)} = \frac{\text{SI } (\mu\text{g/ml})}{1{,}000} \times \text{PV (cc)}$$

$$\times \frac{0.693}{\text{Plasma } ^{59}\text{Fe } T_{1/2} \text{ (min)}} \times 60 \times 24.$$

2. The red cell radioiron incorporation is derived by counting 1 cc whole blood samples from Days 1, 4, 7, 10, and 14 along with the standard. The total red cell mass is then measured with ^{51}Cr on Day 14, correcting for ^{59}Fe Compton contributions to the ^{51}Cr window. Thus,

Red cell incorporation (%)

$$= \frac{^{59}\text{Fe cpm/ml blood} \times {}^{51}\text{Cr blood volume} \times 100}{\text{Total } {}^{59}\text{Fe cpm injected}}.$$

In the above formula no corrections are made for F_{cell} ratio since it is the red cell mass itself we have measured with radiochromium rather than the whole blood volume. In a stable hematologic state, a very simple evaluation of red cell incorporation can be made by dividing the ^{59}Fe cpm/ml blood at Day 14 by the ^{59}Fe cpm/ml whole blood at time zero, the latter derived by back-extrapolation of the plasma disappearance curve and correction to a whole blood value.

3. One-minute surface counts are performed with the external detector described over the spleen (posteriorly unless considerably enlarged), liver, precordium, and bone marrow (sacrum, and frequently in children an additional distal femoral marrow site). With a single detector it is necessary to count over individual sites serially, the first set of counts being performed before significant kinetic changes can occur. If available, a much easier and more effective method is to use four separate detectors placed over the four counting sites and recording simultaneously from time of injection (15). Counts are obtained immediately after radio-iron injection over each counting site, then at the 15, 30, 60, 120, and 240 min time points to characterize the early kinetic changes, and subsequently on Days 1, 2, 3, 4, 7, 10, and 14. Each datum point then has background subtracted and is corrected to day zero for ^{59}Fe decay. This value is then divided by the starting count (time zero) for that organ to normalize all areas to the initial activity level when all radioiron was in the plasma.

Interpretation of the ferrokinetic pattern is well documented in other reviews of the technique (16, 17). The normal plasma radioiron clearance half-time is 60–100 min. The normal plasma iron turnover rate is 0.46–0.78 mg/kg/day (27–42 mg/day in the adult), and red cell radio-iron incorporation at Day 14 is 75–95%. The normal external ferrokinetic pattern demonstrates a rapid marrow rise over the first 4 hr which peaks between 4 and 24 hr and falls back to unity by the 4th to 7th day. There is a slight fall in activity over liver, spleen, and to a greater extent precordium over the first 4–24 hr, followed by a progressive rise almost to unity by 14 days. Hypoplastic anemias demonstrate a prolonged plasma radioiron clearance half-time, decreased plasma iron turnover, and markedly decreased or absent red cell radioiron incorporation. There is reduced or absent marrow radioiron rise over the 4–24-hr time period on external counting, with gradual but steady rise of activity over liver and to a lesser extent spleen up to 14 days. Myeloid metaplasia looks somewhat similar, but demonstrates significant amounts of radioiron appearing in red cells, and the spleen and frequently liver counts rise over 24 hr and subsequently fall indicating release of red-cell-tagged radioiron from these organs. Little or no marrow rise is noted in the first 24 hr, however.

Hemosiderosis and hemochromatosis will demonstrate a normal or a prolonged plasma radioiron clearance half-time which, with a high serum iron, results in increased plasma iron turnover, but a moderately low red cell radioiron incorporation. External counting reveals normal marrow uptake and release but considerable fixed deposition of storage iron in liver and occasionally spleen over 14 days. Iron deficiency or hyperplastic states will demonstrate shortened plasma radioiron clearance half-time with a normal or increased plasma iron turnover rate and a high red cell radioiron incorporation, and essentially a normal external counting pattern which generally is slightly accelerated in time.

One does not need to perform a ferrokinetic study with all of its attendant blood and surface counting to document the presence of simple iron deficiency, marrow hyperplasia, etc. The most important applications of this technique are in the evaluation of extramedullary hematopoiesis and intramedullary hemolysis. The former may be most important in determining whether or not to remove the spleen of a patient with a combination of splenic sequestration and splenic hematopoiesis. The latter will be important in determining the relative contributions of intramedullary and extramedullary hemolysis to a hemolytic anemia, particularly where the possibility of splenectomy is being entertained.

Figure 12-5 summarizes the data in one of our ferrokinetic patients, a young boy of 18 months who was of East Indian descent, his mother having thalassemia minor but his father hematologically normal. Severe anemia had been present from the age of 3 months, requiring transfusions every 2 months thereafter. The only physical findings of significance were diminished weight for his age (50th percentile), pallor, and marked hepatosplenomegaly. A normocytic, normochromic anemia was present with reticulocytes 0.5–1.2%, with platelets and white count normal. The bone marrow demonstrated marked erythroid hyperplasia with early megaloblastoid changes. Hemoglobin electrophoresis and an extensive battery of red cell enzymes were all normal, with normal osmotic fragilities pre- and postincubation, and slightly increased autohemolysis with and without glucose. In addition to the diagnostic dilemma in this patient,

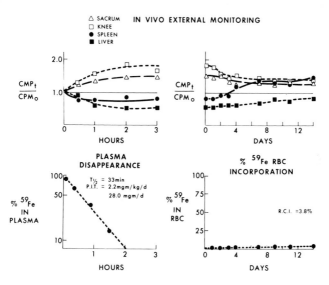

Fig. 12-5. ^{59}Fe ferrokinetic study in child with undiagnosed anemia and hyperplastic marrow. There is good early marrow uptake but incomplete late emptying of tracer indicating ineffective erythropoiesis (intramedullary hemolysis) and to a lesser extent splenic sequestration of the few labeled red blood cells ultimately released into circulation.

major consideration was being given to the possibility that splenectomy might reduce his substantial transfusion requirement.

As seen in Fig. 12-5, the plasma radioiron disappearance half-time was markedly accelerated (33 min). The plasma iron turnover rate was 28.0 mg/day, markedly elevated for a small child. Red cell radioiron incorporation at 14 days was only 3.8%. Surface counting in the first 3 hr demonstrated prompt uptake of tracer in the bone marrow of the sacrum and the knee. Both marrow areas fell only slightly after 24 hr, while the spleen demonstrated a significant rise above unity beyond 72 hr. Thus the iron kinetics study demonstrates predominance of intramedullary hemolysis, with a secondary component of splenic sequestration of young cells just leaving the bone marrow. It is clear that splenectomy would resolve only a minor splenic contribution to his disease. Due to the red cell radioiron incorporation of 3.8%, only 1.1 mg of iron per day will go into peripheral red cell production (0.085 mg/kg/day), resulting in the deposition of almost 27 mg/day of iron in stores, an exceptional iron load which will rapidly build up to a serious degree of hemosiderosis. Although his diagnosis remains unclear, it is suspected to represent an unusual variant of thalassemia major.

Vitamin B_{12} Absorption Studies

The most widely used method of evaluation of vitamin B_{12} absorption is the Schilling test (18). After collection of a 12-hr baseline urine for determination of background radioactivity, 0.007 μCi/kg of [57]Co-vitamin B_{12} is administered orally in the fasting state, and 1 hr later the patient receives 1,000 μg of nonradioactive vitamin B_{12} intramuscularly or subcutaneously. Urine is collected for a period of 24 hr, and then either counted in a large volume counter intact or an aliquot is counted in a well counter, along with a standard to determine the amount of administered tracer displaced into the urine over 24 hr. Normal patients will clear over 10% in the urine in this time period, and patients with pernicious anemia or other types of vitamin B_{12} malabsorption will be found to have less than 7% of the tracer in the urine. In the latter case, the study is repeated after 24–48 hr with one unit intrinsic factor orally at the same time to see if intrinsic factor corrects the absorption defect. If intrinsic factor corrects the absorption defect, the diagnosis is pernicious anemia. In only one patient have we seen apparently classical pernicious anemia fail to demonstrate increased absorption with intrinsic factor. In this instance a significant circulating antibody titer to intrinsic factor was present, and substantially increasing the amount of intrinsic factor did result in increased absorption of the labeled vitamin B_{12}.

Of the eleven children we have studied over the past 5 years, two were from a family with familial pernicious anemia and the remaining nine children had a variety of gastrointestinal problems. Three children with Crohn's disease resulting in extensive small bowel resection all had Schilling tests of less than 4%, whereas two children with Crohn's disease not resected had values of 4 and 19%. The two children with familial pernicious anemia had values of 3 and 4% without intrinsic factor, not rechecked with intrinsic factor.

Other methods of evaluating vitamin B_{12} absorption include quantitating the stool excretion of unabsorbed [57]Co-B_{12}, the 8-hr plasma level of absorbed vitamin B_{12}, the hepatic uptake of labeled vitamin B_{12} several days following administration, and evaluation of total-body retention of orally ingested [58]Co or ^{60}Co-B_{12} by whole-body counting (19). None of these is as widely used as the Schilling test, but the whole-body counting method is by far the most accurate when evaluated at 7 days. The absorbed radiation dose with ^{60}Co-B_{12}, however, is strikingly higher than with the [57]Co-B_{12} (Table 12-1), with substantial radiation to the liver resulting from the long half-life of ^{60}Co and the slow metabolic turnover of vitamin B_{12}.

Other Gastrointestinal Studies

Radioiron absorption can be measured with ^{59}Fe as ferrous citrate administered orally in 1–4 mg of carrier iron. The tracer absorption is best determined by assaying the 7-day stool excretion of unabsorbed radioiron or by total-body counting of retained radioiron at Day 14 (20). The double-isotope method of Saylor and Finch (21) using oral ^{55}Fe and, after 14 days, intravenous ^{59}Fe introduces substantially greater radiation dose to the patient, and potential error in estimating total-body radioiron retention if there is first pass deposition of absorbed iron in the liver as may occur in hemochromatosis or similar iron-loaded states.

Gastrointestinal blood loss is best evaluated with ^{51}Cr, labeling autologous red cells (1.4 μCi/kg) as in the red cell radiochromium study, then collecting stools for 72 hr. Blood loss over this time is then quantitated by comparing stool ^{51}Cr activity with mean blood ^{51}Cr activity from counts at the beginning and the end of the collection period. A normal adult will lose no more than 2 cc of blood per day in the stools by this method, and although specific figures are not available in children, presumably this amount would be scaled down by weight.

Gastrointestinal protein loss is estimated with ^{51}Cr-albumin intravenously, 1.4 μCi/kg, followed by a 96-hr quantitative stool collection, with ^{51}Cr counting against a standard as in the stool blood loss study. In adults, less than 1% of the administered tracer is found in a 96-hr stool collection. Protein-losing gastroenteropathy produces significantly greater amounts of tracer in the stool. The simplest and most effective method of quantitating stool activity is to collect all stools serially or collectively in 1-gallon paint cans, add water up to a fixed total volume in each can, then vigorously agitate to suspend as much of the stool as possible. The counting standard is then made up with a similar amount of water, and the cans are counted in a large volume counter such as the Searle Radiographics Tobor counter.

Bone Marrow Imaging

Bone marrow imaging is an organ imaging technique which is still relatively under-utilized due probably to the diffuse nature of the organ and the difficulties in localizing a specific radiopharmaceutical. Of the radioactive iron isotopes available, only ^{52}Fe (14 μCi/kg) is readily imageable in man using its positron emission, although its 8-hr half-life and the necessity of cyclotron production make it generally unavailable (22). Acid ^{111}In-chloride (30 μCi/kg) appears to be a tracer with significant similarities to iron, binding to the transferrin iron-binding sites, and with as much as 1/3 of the transferrin-bound tracer going to erythroid bone marrow over the next 24–72 hr (23). Although ^{111}In-chloride is widely available, its use in children is limited by significant radiation dose, estimated to be on the order of 1 rad whole body, 4½ rads/mCi to liver, and 3.6 rads/mCi to bone marrow at this administered dose (30 μCi/kg).

Widely available and consequently most useful for bone marrow imaging is ^{99m}Tc-sulfur colloid, 86 μCi/kg, administered 10–15 min be-

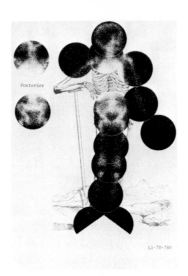

Fig. 12-6. Normal bone marrow distribution in 8-year-old child. Reticuloendothelial element has been imaged with ^{99m}Tc-sulfur colloid and Anger scintillation camera.

fore study. It is estimated that 3–5% of this type of colloidal tracer will localize in bone marrow. By increasing the oscilloscope intensity almost to the blood-flow study level and taking 2-min scintiphotos over appropriate marrow areas, it is possible at completion of a standard liver-spleen scintiphoto study to clearly delineate all the perfused reticuloendothelial marrow. Some colloid preparations, particularly some commercial kits, do not appear to have the same degree of marrow affinity as we have been able to obtain with a standard sulfur colloid method (*24, 25*). The presence of a small amount of stannous ion appears to improve the likelihood of marrow uptake. Although there are hematologic disorders in which a reticuloendothelial label of the marrow does not parallel erythroid and other marrow components (*26*), these are most likely to occur in known disease states such as pure erythroid aplasia, early postirradiation states and some patients with myelofibrosis. With these few exceptions, the radiocolloid marrow image can provide an extremely useful indication of marrow cellularity (*27*), and indirectly of marrow function.

Marrow imaging can also be performed using a whole-body scanner, or in selected regions with a small area scanner, although in our experience scintillation camera images of the marrow are more clearly interpretable in regions of uncertainty. Whichever method of imaging is used, significant problems occur in the region of the lower thoracic and upper lumbar spine, where the dominant activity of the adjacent liver and spleen blocks out marrow visualization.

Figure 12-6 illustrates the normal radiocolloid marrow distribution in a child age 8, demonstrating good axial marrow delineation and evi-

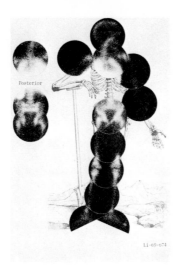

Fig. 12-7. Markedly extended marrow in 10-year-old
child with hemoglobin S-C disease

dence of some peripheral extension as occurs normally in childhood. In general, peripheral extension of marrow to the ends of the extremities is noted at birth and during the first few months of life, with gradual recession of the appendicular marrow during the early 5–15 years of life. Adult marrow distribution without extension beyond the very proximal extremities is seen by age 10 or, at the latest, age 15 in our experience. The presence of anemia or infection over a period of at least several weeks, as illustrated in Fig. 12-7, results in marrow hypertrophy taking the form of peripheral extension, apparently after central marrow has increased its cellularity. Thus, for example, in a child with no known hematologic disorder but the sudden discovery of anemia, demonstration of marked peripheral extension of the marrow would be more suggestive of chronic anemia than an acute process.

Aplastic anemia is associated with virtually total loss of marrow image labeling both with radiocolloid and with radioiron as illustrated in Fig. 12-8. Marrow irradiation at doses above 3,000 rads may also result over several months in loss of radiocolloid (and radioiron) visualization as illustrated in Fig. 12-9. This chronic postirradiation marrow loss is generally considered to be permanent (*28*) although we have found evidence to suggest that marrow recovery can occur under suitable conditions of hematopoietic stress (*29*).

Visualization of solid tumor replacement of the marrow cavity is possible with radiocolloids. This has proved to be a most useful additional parameter in evaluating direct or metastatic tumor spread, par-

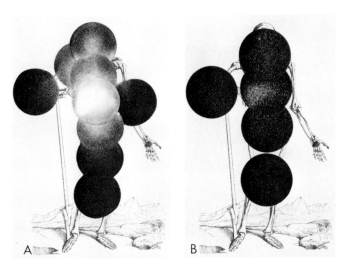

Fig. 12-8. ˮ(A) ^{99m}Tc-sulfur colloid and (B) ^{52}Fe marrow images in child with aplastic anemia, demonstrating complete absence of marrow image with both tracers in disease (performed at Donner Laboratory, University of California, Berkeley).

ticularly in our adult population. Figure 12-10 is the bone marrow study in an 11-year-old girl with Ewing's sarcoma of the proximal right femur, demonstrating displacement of the right femoral marrow by tumor as compared to the normal left femur. Bone scan and standard radiography of the area also demonstrated the presence of the sarcoma, which was subsequently excised and irradiated. Leukemia, particularly acute lymphoblastic leukemia, may be associated with virtually total replacement of normal marrow cellularity by blasts and loss of visualization as illustrated in Fig. 12-11. This is an 8-year-old child with acute lymphoblastic leukemia in exacerbation, associated with anemia and thrombocytopenia, and a densely packed marrow containing 80% blasts. Figure 12-12, on the other hand, is the normal study of a 4½-year-old child with acute lymphoblastic leukemia in remission after 11 months of methotrexate. Marrow cellularity and morphology at this time were normal. Abnormally reduced marrow radiocolloid labeling in blastic leukemia invariably reverts to normal during therapy. When the development of pancytopenia during therapy is associated with normal intensity of marrow labeling, it is almost always the result of aggressive therapy rather than leukemic exacerbation.

Over the past 5 years we have performed bone marrow imaging studies on more than 60 children, covering all the various types of hematologic abnormality mentioned above. The information is often obtained in-

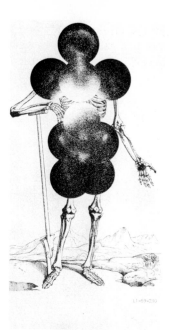

Fig. 12-9. Radiocolloid marrow study in adult with Hodgkin's disease, performed 1 year after total nodal radiotherapy of 4,000 rads. There is striking long-term radioablation of imageable marrow in treatment areas.

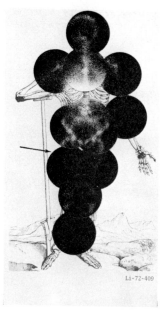

Fig. 12-10. Whole-body marrow study in 11-year-old girl with Ewing's sarcoma involving proximal right femur (arrow). Subtle asymmetry of labeling is noted in proximal femurs. Tumor involvement of axial skeleton in other patients has demonstrated much more prominent defects in marrow labeling.

cidentally in a liver-spleen scintiphoto study and may prove particularly useful in the evaluation of malignant disease, where tumor spread to the marrow may first become evident in the face of normal radiologic studies.

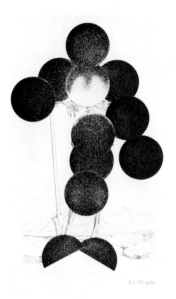

Fig. 12-11. Dense marrow packing by blasts in 8-year-old child with acute lymphoblastic leukemia in exacerbation. Marrow uptake of ^{99m}Tc-sulfur colloid has completely disappeared.

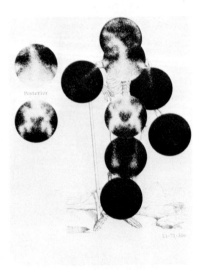

Fig. 12-12. Essentially normal radiocolloid marrow image in 4½-year-old child with acute lymphoblastic leukemia in remission on methotrexate.

Functional Asplenia of Sickle Cell Disease

Imaging of the spleen is covered by Freedman in Chapter 8. However, we have had a particular interest in the functional asplenia of sickle cell disease first described by Pearson, et al in their recent description of this most interesting phenomenon (30). After the first few years of life at most, children with sickle cell disease will generally demonstrate a spleen which is palpably enlarged and yet not visualized by standard radiocolloid techniques. In studies carried out with Louis K. Diamond of our institution, we have observed the same phenomenon (Fig. 12-13). In addition to the absence of visualization of the spleen with ^{99m}Tc-sulfur colloid, this 12-year-old girl demonstrates striking peripheral extension of marrow to the feet consistent with chronic anemia. In the ^{99m}Tc-pertechnetate flow study, marked reduction in splenic perfusion is noted compared to the kidneys, although the 500,000-count blood pool picture demonstrates significant blood content of the spleen. To further evaluate the nature of the functional asplenia by a different technique, autologous red blood cells tagged with ^{51}Cr and heated to 50°C for 1 hr were infused in a standard spleen imaging technique. Scanning 29 hr later demonstrated dominant hepatic uptake with no significant splenic up-

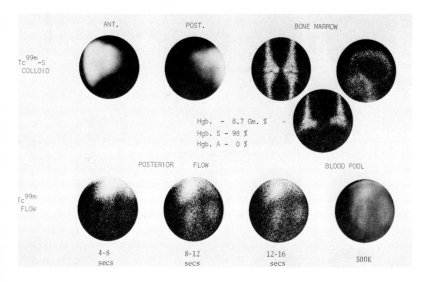

Fig. 12-13. (Upper row) Absence of spleen labeling (functional asplenia) and markedly extended marrow in 12-year-old girl with sickle cell anemia and palpable splenomegaly. (Lower row) ^{99m}Tc-pertechnetate flow study of spleen area shows markedly reduced splenic perfusion compared with kidneys, but definite splenic blood pool at equilibration.

take, as illustrated in Fig. 12-14. This represented a true defect in splenic function rather than a problem with red cell heating, as confirmed by the fact that the blood disappearance half-time of the heat-damaged cells

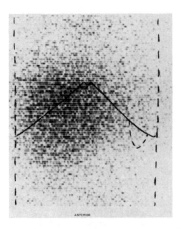

Fig. 12-14. Functional asplenia of sickle cell disease demonstrated with heat-damaged ⁵¹Cr-labeled autologous red blood cells.

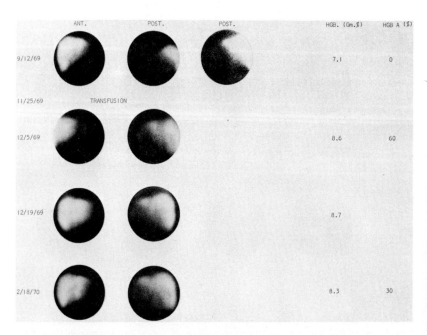

Fig. 12-15. Reversibility of functional asplenia following transfusion of normal blood in 15-year-old boy with sickle cell disease. Spleen image correlates roughly with hemoglobin A level present.

was 213 min, markedly prolonged from normal (42–51 min). Hepatic deposition from overly damaged cells would be associated with rapid blood clearance.

As noted in Fig. 12-15, we were also able to confirm the observation of Pearson, et al (*31*) that transfusion with normal cells resulted in return of spleen visualization, apparently correlated with the hemoglobin A level. The ability to visualize the spleen gradually disappeared as the hemoglobin A level fell over a period of several weeks following transfusion. This fact could also be consistent with the postulate that functional asplenia is not truly a functional defect, but a perfusion defect in the splenic sinusoids, perhaps the result of red cell sickling and sludging. Large numbers of normal red cells might well interrupt the so-called "box carring" of red cells in the microvasculature. Functional asplenia is a fascinating phenomenon in sickle cell disease and might correlate with the incidence of certain infections in these children. As yet, however, the merits of so reducing the functional asplenia do not clearly counterbalance the risks of frequent transfusions simply to maintain a reasonable hemoglobin A level.

Newer Tracer Techniques in Pediatric Hematology

Neutron activation analysis has been explored by several workers in the past as a method of undertaking tracer studies in children without patient radiation exposure. Red cell mass and red cell survival can be studied by labeling of red cells with ^{50}Cr followed by neutron activation of appropriate blood samples (*32*). Ferrokinetic studies may also be performed using ^{58}Fe and neutron activation, although external counting data are of course not obtainable (*33*). Neutron activation has not gained wide use in the past, however, because of the relative lack of availability of high-flux neutron sources in most medical centers (reactors or cyclotrons), and significant complexity of sample handling and tracer quantitation following activation.

Fluorescent excitation analysis, using either monochromatic isotope sources or x-ray sources with or without filtration, can provide a simple method of tracer excitation analysis for a variety of pediatric applications without radiation exposure of the subject (*34, 35*). We have been particularly interested recently in the evaluation of the extracellular fluid volume in children and in adults using nonradioactive sodium bromide administered orally or intravenously (*36, 37*). The amount administered is calculated to produce a plasma bromide concentration of 1–2 mEq/liter after 3–4 hr. The plasma bromide level has been determined by fluorescent excitation using a 2.5 mCi ^{109}Cd exciting source and an 80 mm^2 Si(Li) detector with a 3-mm depletion depth, both collimated to assay approximately a 1 cm^3 region of sensitivity. The 22.10- and 24.99-

keV x-rays of [109]Cd are ideal for excitation of the K-shell electrons of bromine which have a binding energy of 13.48 keV. The subsequent K_α and K_β bromine x-rays of 11.91 and 13.30 keV are easily resolved and readily quantitated by the semiconductor detector. Using a ratio of K_α counts to counts in a defined Compton region, good linearity of quantitation of the bromine is obtained over a concentration range of 0.025–500 mEq/liter.

TABLE 12-4. Comparison of Fluorescent and Chemical Techniques for Bromine Analysis

Patient	Corrected bromide space (liters)		
	Fluorescent	Chemical	% difference
1	3.45	3.62	4.7
2	13.12	11.63	−11.3
3	5.70	5.60	−1.7
4	9.45	9.08	−3.9
5	6.28	5.90	−6.0
6	6.59	7.28	10.5
Avg. diff.			−1.3%
Paired-t (related measures)			0.8 (p > 0.2)
r			0.99 (p < 0.001)

As illustrated in Table 12-4, good correlation is obtained between the corrected bromide spaces in six children as determined by fluorescent excitation, and the corresponding spaces as determined by chemical estimation using Conway's microdiffusion technique (38). Similar excellent correlations were obtained in a group of 11 adults where the nonradioactive tracer was administered orally and [82]Br was administered intravenously (26). Thus determination of the bromide space as an estimate of extracellular fluid volume is now routinely performed in our laboratory using fluorescent excitation analysis, permitting the quantitation of several studies per hour, while the microdiffusion technique previously could be applied only to 5–10 patients per day. We are currently using a 20-mCi [109]Cd source, permitting quantitation of plasma content at these levels with an accuracy of 2% in a 100-sec counting time.

Fluorescent excitation analysis is best applied to tracers of higher atomic weight and to levels at the part per million range or above. Thus it can be used in the evaluation of iodinated radioopaque dyes (35), and it is hoped that we will be able to extend its applicability to such compartment determinations as quantitation of red cell mass using nonradioactive sodium chromate and perhaps estimation of plasma volume using iodinated albumin. Preliminary studies of glomerular filtration rate quantitation in children using nonradioactive iothalamate have recently shown this to be another useful pediatric application of the technique. The principle appears to have very broad clinical applicability in pediatrics once the appropriate nonradioactive tracers and pharmaceuticals have been established for various physiologic and compartment measurements.

Summary

This paper has reviewed the wide variety of radioisotopic techniques available to pediatricians in hematologic evaluation of their patients, with comments on our own experience with these tracer techniques, and an indication of some new territory in splenic evaluation and nonradioactive tracers which may prove to be of considerable interest in the future. As mentioned previously, the only differences in applying these techniques to the pediatric population, compared with the adult population, lie in the different spectrum of hematologic diseases under consideration in this age group and the greater sensitivity to problems of radiation exposure which the pediatrician and the nuclear medicine physician must have in administering the isotopes in vivo. With these considerations in mind, the usefulness of such radioisotopic techniques in the evaluation of pediatric hematologic disease remains unquestionable. The summary in Table 12-1 of the radiopharmaceuticals and the radiation doses associated with the various procedures may be helpful in deciding which procedures should be used to provide the minimum associated risk. It is hoped in the future that fluorescent excitation techniques will replace at least some of the radioisotope techniques, obviating all considerations of patient irradiation in such instances.

Acknowledgments

This work has been supported in part by funds from the Cancer Research Coordinating Committee of the University of California. We appreciate greatly the cooperation of Louis K. Diamond and the Pediatric Hematology Services of the University of California Hospitals and Clinics, and the San Francisco General Hospital, in referring interesting patients for study. The fluorescent excitation work has been possible through provision of a Si(Li) detector by the KeVex Corporation, and the assistance of Leon Kaufman, Malcolm A. Holliday, and Carol Jane Wilson. We are grateful also for the long hours of excellent technical assistance provided by June Ohara, Evelyn Garner, and Jennifer Brunn.

References

1. Seltzer RA, Kereiakes JG, Saenger EL: Radiation exposure from radioisotopes in pediatrics. *N Engl J Med* 271: 84–90, 1964

2. Kereiakes JG, Wellman HN, Tieman J, et al: Radiopharmaceutical dosimetry in pediatrics. *Radiology* 90: 925–930, 1968

3. TOWSON J: The radiation dosimetry of a short-lived radiopharmaceutical acidic indium-113m. *Aust Radiol* 14: 94–100, 1970

4. KEREIAKES JG, WELLMAN HN, SIMMONS G, et al: Radiopharmaceutical dosimetry in pediatrics. *Semin Nucl Med* 2: 316–327, 1972

5. GREENFIELD MA, LANE RG: Radioisotope dosimetry. In *Nuclear Medicine.* Blahd WH, ed, New York, McGraw-Hill, 2nd ed, 1971, pp 120–121

6. FAIRBANKS VF, TAUXE WN: Plasma and erythrocyte volumes in obesity, polycythemia, and related conditions. In *Compartments, Pools and Spaces in Medical Physiology,* Bergner P-EE, Lushbaugh CC, eds, AEC Symoposium Series 11, CONF-661010, Oak Ridge, Tenn, USAEC, 1967, pp 283–298

7. ALBERT SN: Blood volume. In *Nuclear Medicine.* Blahd WH, ed, New York, McGraw-Hill, 2nd ed, 1971, pp 593–619

8. KORUBIN V, MAISEY MN, MCINTYRE, PA: Evaluation of technetium-labeled red cells for determination of red cell volume in man. *J Nucl Med* 13: 760–762, 1972

9. CLINE MJ, BERLIN NI: The red cell chromium elution rate in patients with some hematologic disorders. *Blood* 21: 63–69, 1963

10. ASTER RH, JANDL JH: Platelet sequestration in man. I. Methods. *J Clin Invest* 43: 843–855, 1964

11. HARKER LA, FINCH CA: Thrombokinetics in man. *J Clin Invest* 48: 963–974, 1969

12. MCMILLAN R, SCOTT JL: Leukocyte labeling with ^{51}Chromium. I. Technic and results in normal subjects. *Blood* 32: 738–754, 1968

13. CARTWRIGHT GE, ATHENS JW, WINTROBE MM: The kinetics of granulopoiesis in normal man. *Blood* 24: 780–803, 1964

14. HERSEY P: The separation and ^{51}Chromium labeling of human lymphocytes with in vivo studies of survival and migration. *Blood* 38: 360–371, 1971

15. POLLYCOVE M, MORTIMER R: The quantitative determination of iron kinetics and hemoglobin synthesis in human subjects. *J Clin Invest* 40: 753–782, 1961

16. POLLYCOVE M: Iron metabolism and kinetics. *Semin Hematol* 3: 235–298, 1966

17. HOSAIN F, MARSAGLIA G, FINCH CA: Blood ferrokinetics in normal man. *J Clin Invest* 46: 1–9, 1967

18. SCHILLING RF: Diagnosis of pernicious anemia and other vitamin B_{12} malabsorbtion syndromes with radioactive B_{12}. In *Nuclear Medicine.* Blahd WH, ed, New York, McGraw-Hill, 2nd ed, 1971, pp 444–447

19. REIZENSTEIN PG, CRONKITE EP, COHN SH: Measurement of absorption of vitamin B_{12} by whole-body gamma spectrometry. *Blood* 18: 95–101, 1961

20. PRICE DC, COHN SH, WASSERMAN LR, et al: The determination of iron absorption and loss by whole body counting. *Blood* 20: 517–531, 1962

21. SAYLOR L, FINCH CA: Determination of iron absorption using two isotopes of iron. *Am J Physiol* 172: 372–376, 1953

22. ANGER HO, VAN DYKE D: Human bone marrow distribution shown in vivo by iron-52 and the positron scintillation camera. *Science* 144: 1587–1589, 1964

23. LILIEN DL, BERGER HG, ANDERSON DP, et al: ^{111}Indium-chloride: a new agent for bone marrow imaging. *J Nucl Med* 14: 184–186, 1973

24. STERN HS, MCAFEE JG, SUBRAMANIAN G: Preparation, distribution and utilization of technetium-99m-sulfur colloid. *J Nucl Med* 7: 665–675, 1966

25. LARSON JM, BENNETT LR: Human serum albumin as a stabilizer for ^{99m}Tc-sulfur suspension. *J Nucl Med* 10: 294–295, 1969

26. VAN DYKE D, SHKURKIN C, PRICE D, et al: Differences in distribution of erythropoietic and reticuloendothelial marrow in hematologic disease. *Blood* 30: 364–374, 1967

27. HILL DR, PRICE DC, KANE LJ, et al: Effects of single dose and of fractionated radiation on rabbit bone marrow. *Radiology* 106: 695–698, 1973

28. SYKES MP, SAVEL H, CHU FCH, et al: Long-term effects of therapeutic irradiation upon bone marrow. *Cancer* 17: 1144–1148, 1964

29. PRICE DC, BENAK SB, JR.: Marrow radioablation in man including evidence of recovery with hematopoietic stress. *J Nucl Med* 11: 353, 1970

30. PEARSON HA, SPENCER RP, CORNELIUS EA: Functional asplenia in sickle-cell anemia. *N Engl J Med* 281: 923–926, 1969

31. PEARSON HA, CORNELIUS EA, SCHWARTZ AD, et al: Transfusion-reversible functional asplenia in young children with sickle-cell anemia. *N Engl J Med* 283: 334–337, 1970

32. DONALDSON GWK, JOHNSON PF, TOTHILL P, et al: Red cell survival time in man measured by ^{50}Cr and activation analysis. *Br Med J* 2: 585–587, 1968

33. LOWMAN JT, KRIVIT W: New in vivo tracer method with the use of non-radioactive isotopes and activation analysis. *J Lab Clin Med* 61: 1042–1048, 1963

34. KAUFMAN L, NELSON J, PRICE D, et al: Some applications of Si(Li) detectors to clinical problems. *IEEE Trans Nucl Sci* NS-20: 402–410, 1973

35. KAUFMAN L, PRICE DC, eds: *Semiconductor Detectors in Medicine,* CONF-730321, Oak Ridge, Tenn, USAEC, 1973

36. KAUFMAN L, WILSON CJ: Determination of extracellular fluid volume by fluorescent excitation analysis of bromine. *J Nucl Med* 14: 812–815, 1973

37. PRICE DC, KAUFMAN L, PIERSON RN, JR.: Estimation of the extracellular fluid space in man by fluorescent excitation analysis of bromide: comparison with the radiobromide technique. In preparation

38. CHEEK DB: Estimation of the bromide space with a modification of Conway's method. *J Appl Physiol* 5: 639–644, 1953

Discussion

Richard A. Wetzel (William Beaumont Hospital, Detroit, Mich.): What do you use for normal values for pediatric blood volumes?

Dr. Price: While there is no good reference for these values at the present time, it would appear that 78–84 cc/kg for normal newborns is probably reasonable. This then would decrease until normal adult values of 60–76 cc/kg, depending upon sex, body habitus, etc.

David L. Gilday (Hospital for Sick Children, Toronto, Ontario): In the neonate Robert Usher reported total blood volumes as approximately 100 cc/kg in normals, but there is no information for the group between neonates and adults.

[Editor's note: Usher, Shephard, and Lind (The blood volume of the newborn infant and placental transfusion. *Acta Paediatr Scand* 52: 497–512, 1963) actually reported total blood volumes by ^{131}I-human serum albumin dilution for prematures at 108 cc/kg and normal newborns at 78 cc/kg, with venous hematocrits of 48%. (See Appendix, Table A-8.)]

Chapter **13**

In Vitro Studies: Digoxin

Jerold M. Lowenstein

Radioimmunoassay (RIA) makes it possible to measure nanogram and picogram quantities of important substances in body fluid. Within the past few years, there has been an enormous increase in the use of radioimmunoassay in pediatrics. From January to June 1972 there were articles in *Pediatrics* and *Pediatric Research* based on results of radioimmunoassay of the following: growth hormone (HGH), insulin, FSH, LH, LRH, prolactin, thyroid and parathyroid hormones, testosterone, vitamin B_{12}, and digoxin.

Radioimmunoassay procedures require a labeled antigen, an antibody or specific binding protein, and a method for separating the bound from the unbound antigen. Although the principle is simplicity itself, with a standard curve relating percent bound to concentration of the material to be measured, many difficulties can enter the assay from any of these three components. For example, antigen may be damaged by the labeling procedure and react poorly with antibody; antibody may not be sufficiently specific and may bind to related molecules present in the serum; a separation technique (e.g., charcoal) may not only separate the bound from the free material but also separate the antigen from its antibody. These problems, the problems of immunizing animals, and volumes of others are set down in agonizing detail in the proceedings of the many symposia devoted to this subject during the past few years including the conferences on protein and polypeptide hormones at Liège (*1, 2*).

While these developmental struggles are unavoidable in a research endeavor, the availability of handy commercial kits now makes it possible for most departments of nuclear medicine or clinical laboratories to do RIAs of the more common variety (T_4, B_{12}, insulin, Australia antigen, digoxin) without the headaches of immunizing rabbits, caring for them, and finding out all the things that can go wrong with an assay created de novo.

In particular, the availability of an ^{125}I-labeled digoxin analog and digoxin antibody in kit form makes serum digoxin measurement a routine laboratory test. Kaplan discusses RIA techniques in endocrinology in Chapter 14. I will dwell on the digoxin RIA as an example of methods and problems covering specific applications to pediatrics.

History

Since Withering began its clinical use, digitalis dose has been a complex medical problem in children and adults because of the low toxic-to-therapeutic ratio and the high mortality in heart-damaged patients when the dose is either too high or two low (3). Neither clinical judgment nor electrocardiographic signs have proved adequate for assessing toxicity. Radioisotopes provided for the first time the requisite sensitivity for measuring blood levels of cardiac glycosides. The earliest work was done by administering [3]H- or ^{14}C-labeled glycosides to patients and measuring plasma activity (4). Subsequently this writer developed a method for measuring plasma levels based on inhibition of ^{86}Rb uptake by red cells (5, 6). In 1967 Butler and Chen succeeded in producing digoxin-specific antibodies in rabbits, thereby making RIA feasible (7), and Smith and coworkers have applied this assay to clinical problems (8).

Technique

To point up some of the complexities of RIA, neither the antigen used for immunizing animals nor the "labeled antigen" in the assay is digoxin, in the most commonly used method. Digoxin is not normally immunogenic; to make it so, it must be coupled (as hapten) to another molecule, usually bovine serum albumin, and the complex used to immunize rabbits. Tritium and ^{14}C-digoxin are used successfully as labeled antigens, but this requires liquid scintillation counting. To use the simpler and more available gamma counting, it is necessary to substitute a digoxin analog, 3-O-succinyl tryosine digoxigenin, labeled with ^{125}I, which can be shown to behave almost identically with digoxin in the assay (Fig. 13-1) (but not in vivo, as unpublished work by this investigator has shown).

In the clinical assay, to a small amount (about 50 μl) of patient's serum in buffer, is added: first the ^{125}I-digoxigenin and then a fixed amount of digoxin antiserum; this is incubated 30 min at room temperature; finally a fixed amount of Dextran-coated charcoal is added, the tube centrifuged, and the supernatant (bound fraction) decanted and

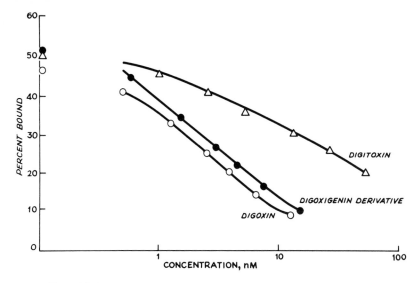

Fig. 13-1. Comparison of ability of digoxin, digitoxin, and 3-O-succinyl digoxigenin tyrosine to displace 3-O-succinyl digoxigenin tyrosine (^{125}I) from antibody binding site.

counted in a scintillation counter. Figure 13-1 shows a typical standard curve, plotted as percent bound versus concentration of digoxin. It also shows the parallelism of displacement by the digoxigenin derivative, and the weak cross reaction with digitoxin.

Clinical Use

Considering the number of drugs and salts known to have either potentiating or inhibiting effects on digitalis as used clinically, it has been surprising how little "gray area" there has been between toxic and non-toxic serum levels. Smith, et al, for instance, found in adults that roughly 85% of those below 2 ng/ml were clinically nontoxic, and roughly 85% of those above 2 ng/ml were clinically toxic (8). The general experience is that levels greater than 3 ng/ml are almost always associated with toxicity and those under 2 ng/ml rarely (9). There is accumulating data confirming the clinical experience of pediatric cardiologists that larger doses of digoxin on a weight basis are both needed and tolerated. Rogers, et al (10) found in neonates and infants that the substantially higher doses being used resulted in higher mean serum levels (2.0 ng/ml compared with 1.3 ng/ml in adults) without signs of intoxication. Soyka (11) studied three age groups and found higher average doses per kilogram and higher mean serum levels in younger children (Table 13-1).

TABLE 13-1. Digoxin Dose and Serum Levels in Children (Ref. *11*)

Age	Digoxin dose (μg/kg)	Mean serum digoxin (ng/ml)
6 mo–2 yr	20	3.2
2–5 yr	16	2.2
5–12 yr	9	1.8

Recent studies have suggested an "epidemic" of digoxin toxicity (8 –20% of hospitalized patients) with an average mortality of 22% (*3*). Other surveys have emphasized the variables of GI absorption (*12*), brand of digoxin (*13*), and patient compliance (i.e., not taking the medicine) (*14*).

For all these reasons, it is essential to have an objective measure of the adequacy of digitalization, particularly in infants and children. RIA, which is fast, accurate, and requires only small amounts of blood, is becoming indispensable in clinical cardiology.

Summary

Radioimmunoaasay is an ideal application of nuclear medicine to pediatrics, making it possible to measure nanogram and picogram quantities of compounds in the serum. The digoxin RIA is illustrative of the problems and applications of the technique. Both dose and serum levels of digoxin are higher (on a weight basis) in infants and children than in adults. Because of the narrow therapeutic range of digoxin and its dangerous toxicity, and with the variability introduced with age, metabolic factors, absorption, and compliance, digoxin RIA has become indispensable to the cardiologist.

References

1. MARGOULIES M, ed: *Protein and Polypeptide Hormones.* Amsterdam, Excerpta Medica, 1968

2. MARGOULIES M, GREENWOOD FC, eds: *Structure-Activity Relationships of Protein and Polypeptide Hormones.* Amsterdam, Excerpta Medica, 1971

3. BELLER GA, SMITH TW, ABELMANN WH, et al: Digitalis intoxication—a prospective clinical study with serum level correlations. *N Engl J Med* 284: 989–997, 1971

4. DOHERTY JE: The clinical pharmacology of digitalis glycosides: a review. *Am J Med Sci* 255: 382–414, 1968

5. LOWENSTEIN JM: A method for measuring plasma levels of digitalis glycosides. *Circulation* 31: 228–233, 1965

6. LOWENSTEIN JM, CORRILL EM: An improved method for measuring plasma and tissue concentrations of digitalis glycosides. *J Lab Clin Med* 67: 1048–1052, 1966

7. BUTLER VP, CHEN JP: Digoxin-specific antibodies. *Proc Natl Acad Sci* 57: 71–78, 1967

8. SMITH TW, BUTLER VP, HABER E: Determination of therapeutic and toxic serum digoxin concentrations by radioimmunoassay. *N Engl J Med* 281: 1212–1216, 1969

9. DOHERTY JE: Serum digitalis levels: clinical use. *Ann Intern Med* 74: 787–789, 1971

10. ROGERS MC, WILLERSON JT, GOLDBLATT A, et al: Serum digoxin concentrations in the human fetus, neonate and infant. *N Engl J Med* 287: 1010–1013, 1972

11. SOYKA LF: Clinical pharmacology of digoxin. *Pediatr Clin North Am* 19: 241–256, 1972

12. HEIZER WD, SMITH TW, GOLDFINGER SE: Absorption of digoxin in patients with malabsorption syndromes. *N Engl J Med* 285: 257–259, 1971

13. WAGNER JG, CHRISTENSEN M, SAKMAR E, et al: Equivalence lack in digoxin plasma levels. *JAMA* 224: 199–204, 1973

14. WEINTRAUB M, AU WYW, LASAGNA L: Compliance as a determinant of serum digoxin concentration. *JAMA* 224: 481–485, 1973

Discussion

Michael A. Lawson (Good Samaritan Hospital, Phoenix, Ariz.): When performing digoxin levels on an emergency basis, do you run a standard curve or do you use a previously established curve?

Dr. Lowenstein: If it is later the same day, we use the earlier standard curve, but one should be run on each day that an assay is performed.

Philip O. Alderson (Mallinckrodt Institute of Radiology, St. Louis, Mo.): What levels of digoxin are toxic in children?

Dr. Lowenstein: Clinical toxicity is rarely seen below 3 ng/ml and may not be evident up to 4 ng/ml, in contrast with adults, in whom 85% manifest toxicity above 2 ng/ml.

Gerald DeNardo (University of California, Davis, Calif.): With a constant antibody to digoxigenin, there seems to be a constant relationship between the standard curve for digoxin and the curve of cross-reaction with digitoxin. If this relationship is reliable, couldn't one perform the digoxin assay, and with appropriate correction factors predict the level of either glycoside?

Dr. Lowenstein: For a given antibody, digoxin-digitoxin cross-reactivity is fairly constant and runs about 10-1. Therapeutic digitoxin levels also run about ten times as high as digoxin levels, so this assay is sufficient for measuring digitoxin, although not as sensitive as one based on a specific digitoxin antibody. Once the cross-reaction is established (as in Fig. 13-1), that fixed ratio can be used to determine digitoxin levels while using that antibody. With a new antibody, the ratio might change and must be checked with digitoxin standards.

Chapter **14**

In Vitro Studies: Endocrinological

Selna L. Kaplan

The availability of sensitive radioimmunoassays for protein and steroid hormones (*1–7*) which require small volumes of plasma (50 μl–1 ml) have provided a means to assess a variety of endocrine disorders in children. All radioimmunoassay procedures are based on the interaction of radioactive-labeled and unlabeled hormone with a hormone-specific antiserum. Iodine-131 or ^{125}I are used for labeling protein hormones and ^{3}H for steroid hormones.

For example, the binding of ^{131}I-hGH with antiserum to human growth hormone (hGH) is displaced by the addition of increasing amounts of unlabeled hGH to establish a standard reference curve for the assay (Fig. 14-1). The percent displacement of binding induced by diluted serum or urine samples is then read off the standard curve and multiplied by the sample dilution to obtain the concentration of the hormone per milliliter of plasma.

Growth Hormone (GH)

Random levels of GH are often low in normal children and are indistinguishable from levels in children who have GH deficiency (*8*). This has necessitated the use of a variety of agents which stimulate the release of GH, not all of which have a significant physiologic role. The tests used most frequently, with the peak time for response in each, are shown in Table 14-1.

A specific physiologic stimulator of GH release is sleep. With the onset of deep sleep a significant release of GH occurs which is related to sleep phase, not time of day. In contrast with other stimuli, GH release

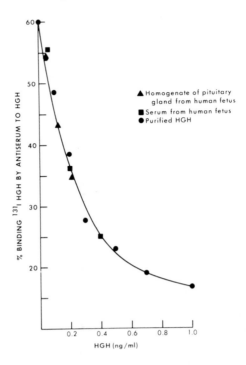

Fig. 14-1. Standard curve for radioimmunoassay of hGH. Percent binding of labeled hGH to specific antibody to hGH is on ordinate and concentration of unlabeled hGH is on abscissa. Decreased binding of ¹³¹I-hGH to antisera is induced by increasing concentrations of unlabeled hGH.

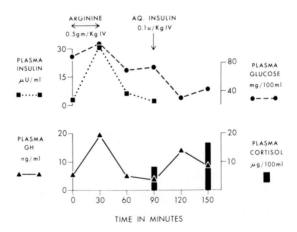

Fig. 14-2. Hormonal response to arginine-insulin stimulation tests. Plasma growth hormone response to arginine infusion and insulin-induced hypoglycemia is indicated by triangles in lower half. Solid bars indicate plasma cortisol response to insulin-induced hypoglycemia.

TABLE 14-1. Agents Affecting the Release of Growth Hormone

Stimulus	Dose	Peak time for response (min)
Insulin-induced hypoglycemia	0.1 U/kg i.v.	30–60
Arginine	0.5 gm/kg infused over 30 min	45–60
L-dopa	200–500 mg p.o.	30–60
Glucagon	15 μg/kg i.v.	5–15
	0.5 mg i.m.	30–45
Exercise		30–45
Sleep	Stage 3–4	60–120

following sleep is not suppressed by glucose, cortisone, or sedatives (9, 10). Unless sampling is performed with electroencephalographic patterns of sleep, peak time for sampling may be inaccurate and result in blunted GH responses. In the child, the mean maximal response to any of these stimuli is 12.5 ng/ml. Any rise above 7 ng/ml is usually indicative of normal GH secretion, whereas values less than 3 ng/ml in response to more than one stimulus are consistent with GH deficiency (5, 11).

The observation of discrepancies in GH responsiveness to a single stimulus in approximately 30% of children has led to the use of a double-barreled test: arginine infusion followed by insulin-induced hypoglycemia. With this combination, not only GH release but ACTH function can be assessed, as reflected by the plasma cortisol response to hypoglycemia (Fig. 14-2).

Thyroid Function

Both triiodothyronine (T_3) and thyroxine (T_4) can now be measured by specific radioimmunoassay methods. The normal range in children of T_4 is 3.5–8.0 μg% and of T_3 100–200 ng/ml. One important application of the measurement of T_3 has been in the identification of individuals with T_3 thyrotoxicosis. These patients have clinical symptomatology consistent with hyperthyroidism, normal T_4 levels, but elevated concentrations of serum T_3 (12). An inborn error of thyroid metabolism has been described as well in clinically euthyroid patients, which is associated with goiter, low-to-borderline levels of T_4 and elevated T_3.

The measurement of thyroid-stimulating hormone (TSH) is useful in the evaluation of abnormalities of thyroid function. In primary hypothyroidism, the concentration of plasma TSH is 50–500 μU/ml (normal 2–8 μU/ml). In most instances, the measurement of TSH is confirmatory of clinical and laboratory evidence of low levels of thyroxine. In some pa-

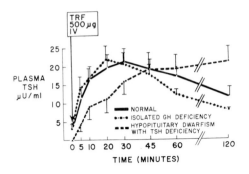

tients, the concentration of plasma TSH may be the prime evidence for an impending hypothyroid state, as illustrated by children with thyroid remnants or ectopic thyroid glands. In these patients, the PBI and T₄ are within the normal range but the plasma TSH is markedly elevated. Similar findings have been observed in some patients with Hashimoto's thyroiditis. Plasma TSH can also be used to assess the adequacy of replacement and suppression therapy postoperatively in patients with thyroid carcinoma.

The regulation of the secretion of hormones from the anterior pituitary is modulated by stimulatory and inhibitory hormones released by the hypothalamus. The differentiation of primary from secondary hypothyroidism can now be determined by the plasma TSH response to synthetic thyrotropin-releasing factor (TRF). This hormone, identical to that present in the hypothalamus of humans and animals, induces a rapid rise in TSH in individuals with an intact pituitary gland (*13, 14*). The TSH response of most children with hypopituitarism and secondary hypothyroidism is comparable to that of normal children and those with isolated GH deficiency (Fig. 14-3). A comparable release of prolactin in each group is induced by administration of TRF (*15, 16*). This indicates that most patients with idiopathic hypopituitarism have an intact pituitary gland but a deficiency in the release and/or synthesis of hypophysiotropic hormones. Thus they have secondary hypopituitarism or hypophysiotropic hypopituitarism.

Abnormalities of Sexual Development

Our laboratory and others have established that changes occur in the concentration of plasma FSH, LH, and sex steroids during puberty

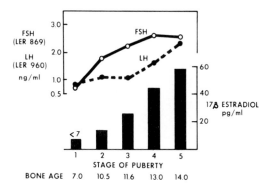

Fig. 14-4. Hormonal changes during puberty in female. Plasma LH and FSH at different stages of puberty are shown in upper section and plasma estradiol (pg/ml) as bars in lower half.

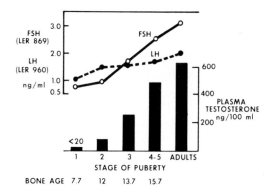

Fig. 14-5. Hormonal changes during male puberty. Plasma LH and FSH increases with progression of puberty as indicated in upper section. Plasma testosterone (ng/100 ml) indicated by bar graph, shows sharp increment with advancement of puberty.

(*17–19*). Plasma LH and FSH are also measurable in prepubertal individuals.

In the female, onset of breast budding occurs at a mean age of 11.2 years with a range of 9–13 years. The mean duration of puberty from breast budding to menses is 2.3 years. Plasma FSH rises during the early stages of puberty, whereas plasma LH increases slowly during puberty in the female (Fig. 14-4). Estradiol shows a concordant rise from a concentration of less than 10 pg/ml* prepubertally to significant increases at midpuberty to 25 pg/ml (*17*).

In the male, mean age at onset of puberty is 12 years with a mean range of 10–15 years. The earliest changes are thinning and increased vascularity of scrotal skin with subsequent testicular enlargement. Plasma

* pg = picogram.

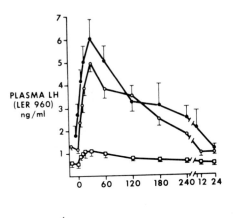

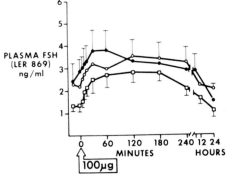

Fig. 14-6. Plasma LH and FSH response to 100 µg of synthetic LRF of prepubertal children (squares), pubertal males (open circles), and adult males (closed circles) is shown. Note meager LH response of prepubertal children with marked increase in responsiveness with onset of puberty. Adult males have response greater than that of pubertal males. Plasma FSH response to LRF shows no significant change with onset of puberty, as noted in lower section.

LH rises before FSH during puberty in the male (Fig. 14-5). Testosterone rises slightly in early stages of puberty but is significantly elevated by mid-puberty (248 ng/%) (*18*).

In patients with primary hypogonadism associated with sex chromosomal abnormalities, increased levels of plasma LH and FSH are present even in the young prepubertal child (2 months to 1 year of age) and provide early assessment of adequacy of gonadal function.

The recent synthesis of the hypothalamic-luteinizing releasing factor (LRF) (*20*), which induces the release of FSH and LH, has provided a further means of evaluation of the functional state of the hypothalamic-pituitary-gonadal system. From our own studies (*21*) and those of Job and associates (*22*), it is evident that the prepubertal child has a lesser rise in LH following LRF than the pubertal or adult individual, but that the FSH response is similar in all groups pre- and post-puberty (Fig. 14-6). In the patient with hypogonadotropic hypogonadism, decreased or absent LH and FSH responses are observed following LRF administration (21–23). These data suggest that the degree of prior exposure of the pituitary to circulating endogenous LRF may affect the gonadotropic response to the LRF stimulation test, in marked contrast to the results obtained following stimulation with the other hypothalamic-releasing factor, TRF, in these same patients.

In patients with delayed adolescence who have no signs, or minimal signs, of pubertal development, the response to LRF may provide evidence of an intact functioning mature hypothalamus and pituitary gland. In these "late prepubertal" patients, despite lack of physical signs of puberty, the basal levels of FSH, LH, testosterone, and the response to LRF were consistent with the onset of puberty (23).

In children with premature thelarche, or in those with idiopathic sexual precocity, plasma estradiol shows a slight-to-moderate elevation, consistent with the degree of sexual development. In girls with ovarian tumors or a feminizing tumor of the adrenal, marked elevations in plasma estradiol are observed (17). Preliminary evidence in our laboratory suggests that the response to LRF may permit differentiation of young patients with premature breast development from those with early sexual precocity. In the former, the plasma LH is that of a prepubertal child, and in the latter a pubertal plasma LH response is observed.

Adrenal Disorders

In children, particularly in the early neonatal period, the measurement of plasma 17-OH progesterone may be critical in the early diagnosis of congenital virilizing adrenal hyperplasia. This hormone, a precursor in the biosynthetic pathway for cortisol, is markedly elevated in patients with the adrenogenital syndrome (24–26). It is metabolized and excreted in the urine primarily as pregnanetriol, which is markedly elevated in this disorder.

Plasma 17-OH progesterone is also elevated during gestation and at term. The levels in cord blood of normal newborns are high (1,000 ng/100 ml), but decrease rapidly to levels less than 50 ng/100 ml by 12 hr. They remain in this range throughout childhood. In patients with virilizing adrenal hyperplasia, the levels are 50–200-fold above normal. The concentration of 17-OH progesterone is more than 1,000 ng/100 ml in all young patients with this disorder (26). It is thus possible for the diagnosis and therapeutic management of this disorder to use small samples of blood obtained by heel-stick, which negates the need for 24-hr urinary collections.

References

1. BERSON SA, YALOW RS: Immunoassay of protein hormones. In *The Hormones,* Pincus G, Thimann KV, Astwood EB, eds, vol 4, New York, Academic Press, 1964, pp 557–630

2. POTTS JT, SHERWOOD LM, O'RIORDAN JLH, et al: Radioimmunoassay of polypeptide hormones. *Adv Intern Med* 13: 183–240, 1967

3. MURPHY BEP: Some studies of the protein-binding of steroids and their application to the routine micro and ultramicro measurement of various steroids in body fluids by competitive protein-binding radioassay. *J Clin Endocrinol Metab* 27: 973–990, 1967

4. ABRAHAM GE, ODELL WD: Solid-phase radioimmunoassay of serum estradiol-17β: a semi-automated approach. In *Immunologic Methods in Steroid Determination,* Peron FG, Caldwell BV, eds, New York, Appleton-Century-Crofts, 1970, pp 87–112

5. YOULTON R, KAPLAN SL, GRUMBACH MM: Growth and growth hormone: IV. Limitations of the growth hormone response to arginine in the assessment of growth hormone deficiency in children. *Pediatrics* 43: 989–1004, 1969

6. BURR IM, SIZONENKO PC, KAPLAN SL, et al: Hormonal changes in puberty. I. Correlation of serum luteinizing hormone and follicle stimulating hormone with stages of puberty, testicular size, and bone age in normal boys. *Pediatr Res* 4: 25–35, 1970

7. SIZONENKO PC, BURR IM, KAPLAN SL, et al: Hormonal changes in puberty. II. Correlation of serum luteinizing hormone and follicle stimulating hormone with stages of puberty and bone age in normal girls. *Pediatr Res* 4: 36–45, 1970

8. KAPLAN SL: Growth hormone secretion and the evaluation of growth retardation in children. In *Laboratory Tests in Diagnosis and Investigation of Endocrine Function,* Escamilla RF, ed, 2nd ed, Philadelphia, FA Davis, 1971, pp 35–44

9. TAKAHASHI Y, KIPNIS DM, DAUGHADAY WH: Growth hormone secretion during sleep. *J Clin Invest* 47: 2079–2090, 1968

10. GLICK SM: The regulation of growth hormone secretion. In *Frontiers in Neuroendocrinology 1969,* Ganong WF, Martini L, eds, New York, Oxford University Press, 1969, pp 141–182

11. ROOT AW, ROSENFIELD RL, BONGIOVANNI AM, et al: The plasma growth hormone response to insulin-induced hypoglycemia in children with retardation of growth. *Pediatrics* 39: 844–852, 1967

12. CHOPRA IJ, HO RS, LAM R: An improved radioimmunoassay of triiodothyronine in serum: its application to clinical and physiological studies. *J Lab Clin Med* 80: 729–739, 1972

13. COSTOM BH, GRUMBACH MM, KAPLAN SL: Effect of thyrotropin releasing factor on serum thyroid-stimulating hormone. An approach to distinguishing hypothalamic from pituitary forms of idiopathic hypopituitary dwarfism. *J Clin Invest* 50: 2219–2225, 1971

14. JACOBS LS, SNYDER PJ, WILBER JF, et al: Increased serum prolactin after administration of synthetic thyrotropin releasing hormone (TRH) in man. *J Clin Endocrinol Metab* 33: 996–998, 1971

15. KAPLAN SL, GRUMBACH MM, FRIESEN HG, et al: Thyrotropin-releasing factor (TRF) effect on secretion of human pituitary prolactin and thyrotropin in children and in idopathic hypopituitary dwarfism: Further evidence for hypophysiotropic hormone deficiencies. *J Clin Endocrinol Metab* 35: 825–830, 1972

16. FOLEY TP, OWINGS J, HAYFORD JT, et al: Serum thyrotropin responses to synthetic thyrotropin-releasing hormone in normal children and hypopituitary patients. *J Clin Invest* 51: 431–437, 1972

17. JENNER MR, KELCH RP, KAPLAN SL, et al: Hormonal changes in puberty: IV. Plasma estradiol, LH, and FSH in prepubertal children, pubertal females, and in precocious puberty, premature thelarche, hypogonadism, and in a child with a feminizing ovarian tumor. *J Clin Endocrinol Metab* 34: 521–530, 1972

18. AUGUST GP, GRUMBACH MM, KAPLAN SL: Hormonal changes in puberty: III. Correlation of plasma testosterone, LH, FSH, testicular size, and bone age with male pubertal development. *J Clin Endocrinol Metab* 34: 319–326, 1972

19. BLIZZARD RM, JOHANSON A, GUYDA H, et al: Recent developments in the study of gonadotropin secretion in adolescence. In *Adolescent Endocrinology,* Heald FP, Hung W, eds, New York, Appleton-Century-Crofts, 1970, pp 1–42

20. AMOSS M, BURGUS R, BLACKWELL R, et al: Purification, amino acid composition and N-terminus of the hypothalamic luteinizing hormone releasing factor (LRF) of ovine origin. *Biochem Biophys Res Com* 44: 205–210, 1971

21. ROTH JC, KELCH RP, KAPLAN SL, et al: FSH and LH response to luteinizing hormone-releasing factor in prepubertal and pubertal children, adult males and patients with hypogonadotropic and hypergonadotropic hypogonadism. *J Clin Endocrinol Metab* 35: 926–930, 1972

22. JOB JC, GARNIER PE, CHAUSSAIN JL, et al: Elevation of serum gonadotropins (LH-FSH) after releasing hormone (LH-RH) injection in normal children and in patients with disorders of puberty. *J Clin Endocrinol Metab* 35: 473–476, 1972

23. GRUMBACH MM, ROTH JC, KAPLAN SL, et al: Hypothalamic-pituitary regulation of puberty: Evidence and concepts derived from clinical research. In *The Control of the Onset of Puberty,* Grumbach MM, Grave GD, Mayer F, eds, New York, Wiley, 1974, pp 115–166

24. STROTT CA, YOSHIMI T, LIPSETT MB: Plasma progesterone and 17-hydroxyprogesterone in normal men and children with congenital adrenal hyperplasia. *J Clin Invest* 48: 930–939, 1969

25. ATHERDEN SM, BARNES ND, GRANT DB: Circadian variation in plasma 17-hydroxyprogesterone in patients with congenital adrenal hyperplasia. *Arch Dis Childh* 47: 602–604, 1972

26. JENNER MR, GRUMBACH MM, KAPLAN SL, et al: Unpublished data, 1972

Chapter **15**

Clinical Experience in a Children's Hospital

David L. Gilday

The Hospital for Sick Children in Toronto is an 800-bed pediatric hospital which acts as the major referral center for the province of Ontario and is the pediatric teaching hospital for the University of Toronto. In January 1972 a Division of Nuclear Medicine was established within the Department of Radiology. Presently it is made up of a "hot" lab, three clinical laboratory rooms, three offices, and secretarial space. In addition, common facilities are shared with the Radiology Department. The staff consists of a full-time physician, a resident, three technicians, a Women's Auxiliary volunteer, a half-time radiopharmacist, a consultant physicist, and a secretary. The equipment in our division consists of a Picker Dynacamera II-C gamma camera, an Ohio-Nuclear dual 5-in. crystal scanner with minification, a single 3-in. crystal scanner for animal research, and an assortment of probe and well-counting facilities.

Work Load

In our first year, there was a marked increase in the number of studies done per month from 47 to 258. The total for our first year was 1,950 procedures in 1,354 patients. Currently we average 12 procedures per day. Table 15-1 summarizes the workload during the first year. Examination of the central nervous system constituted 56% of our workload because of the active neurosurgical and neurological services in the hospital. Fifty-one percent of all the studies of the brain and cerebral spinal fluid space were abnormal. In the other systems, the abnormality rate varied from a high of 92% in the urinary tract to a low of 4% when

TABLE 15-1. Workload during First Year

Study	No.	Percent abnormal
Brain scans	616	49
Radionuclide angiograms	341	
CSF studies	50	80
CSF shunt studies	94	49
Bone scans	30	77
Radioactive iodine uptakes	83	58
Thyroid scans	72	39
Lung scans	23	80
Liver and spleen scans	79	55
Meckel's diverticulum	24	4
Kidney studies	162	92

searching for Meckel's diverticula. In adult nuclear medicine, it would be unusual to have such a high abnormality rate. This reflects the careful selection of our patients by the clinicians who are naturally cautious in ordering radionuclide studies for children.

The ideal clinical investigation, and our goal, is to use the diagnostic procedure which will offer the most definitive information and thus reduce the number of unnecessary or repetitive procedures. Bone scans, which are more sensitive than the radiological skeletal survey, have begun to replace the latter in the investigation of metastatic disease. In evaluating the renal system, a number of instances occur when the radionuclidic study is the procedure of choice, e.g., in patients allergic to iodine or in severe renal failure who are difficult to examine radiologically. In such instances a ^{99m}Tc-DTPA kidney study is valuable in delineating renal pathology. The kidney study has proved to be a most versatile means of evaluating renal transplants, especially for post-renal obstruction and delineation of renal blood supply.

Brain Studies

The brain scan has become the primary diagnostic procedure in patients suspected of having intracranial pathology and is of proven value in indicating the correct and logical direction of subsequent neurological investigation. To further illustrate the role of nuclear medicine in the daily practice of pediatrics, the following is a detailed analysis of our experience with brain scanning.

Among the commoner symptoms which resulted in brain scans being performed in 1972 were headaches and seizures (Table 15-2). We found that there was a reasonable yield of abnormal studies in patients who presented with either headaches or seizures alone; however, when focal neurological signs were included with headaches or seizures as part

TABLE 15-2.   Positive Brain Scan Yield

Symptom	No.	No. positive
Headaches	54	11+
Headaches and neurological signs	13	9+
Seizures	103	17+
Seizures and neurological signs	8	6+

of the presenting symptom complex, there was an extremely high yield of abnormal brain scans. Among the commoner diagnoses encountered were encephalitis, tumor, subdural hematoma, and cerebral vascular accident.

We examined 56 patients with brain tumors. Ten of these patients had recurrence of a previously diagnosed and treated tumor. The remainder were new and undiagnosed cases. Fifty-four of 56 patients examined had abnormal brain scans (Table 15-3). One interesting feature is that more of our tumors were supratentorial (ST) rather than infratentorial (IT), as was found in a 5-year study in our hospital where 51% of the tumors were supratentorial. Contrary to widely held views, we found that carefully performed delayed (2–4-hr postinjection) brain scans yield good results in medulloblastomas, ependymomas, and craniopharyngiomas.

Abnormalities of cerebral blood flow occur frequently in children; however, unlike adults they are usually not due to cerebral vascular accidents but are associated with hydrocephalus or dural fluid collections (Table 15-4). Of 17 patients with hydrocephalus, only 7 had decreased perfusion to the central portions of each hemisphere indicating the enlarged ventricles. Of 32 patients who had subdural hematomas, 31 had abnormalities in either the cerebral radionuclide angiogram or in the 2-hr delayed brain scan. This delay has decreased the number of false-negative

TABLE 15-3.   Brain Tumors

Histology	No.	No. positive
Astrocytoma (ST)	22	20+
(IT)	5	5+
Medulloblastoma (ST)	5	5+
(IT)	6	6+
Craniopharyngioma	7	7+
Ependymoma	5	5+
Chordoma	1	1+
Pinealoma	1	1+
Lymphosarcoma	1	1+
Tumor type unidentified	3	3+
Total	56	54+

TABLE 15-4. Vascular Problems

Diagnosis	No.	No. positive
Hydrocephalus	17	7+
Subdural hematomas	32	31+
Arterial obstruction	10	9+

TABLE 15-5. Trauma

Diagnosis	No.	No. positive
Skull fracture	7	7+
Craniotomy	10	10+
Contusion—brain	4	4+
Subgaleal hematoma	1	1+
Cephalohematoma	4	4+

studies. Nine of ten arterial obstructions (intracerebral or carotid) had abnormal scans.

Skull trauma often causes brain scan abnormalities (Table 15-5). This is usually considered to be a detriment to the brain scan interpretation of intracranial pathology; however, with the aid of the radionuclide cerebral angiogram, brain contusions, scalp hematomas, and skull fractures can be separated from subdural hematomas.

Lastly, inflammatory lesions are very common. In addition to the usual abnormalities such as the peripheral increase of meningitis focal lesions of subgaleal and intracerebral abscesses, we found an unusual pattern of intracranial inflammation. This pattern was a diffuse increase in radioactivity throughout the cerebral hemispheres obliterating the normal contrast between the vascular anatomy and the brain itself (Fig. 15-1). This was first noted by Conway in 1972 (1). It is most commonly

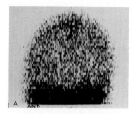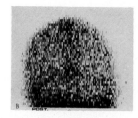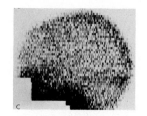

Fig. 15-1. Encephalitis. Routine 3-hr brain scan shows diffuse increase in uptake throughout cerebral hemispheres and cerebellum obliterating normal contrast between vascular anatomy and brain substance. (A) anterior, (B) posterior, and (C) lateral.

TABLE 15-6. Inflammatory Lesions		
Diagnosis	No.	No. positive
Encephalitis	8	6+
Meningitis	6	4+
Subgaleal abscess	3	3+
Cerebral abscess	4	4+
Ventriculitis	1	1+

due to encephalitis or meningitis. Our overall accuracy in delineating and detecting inflammatory lesions was 82% (Table 15-6).

Summary

Our experience indicates that there is a much higher information yield from integrated rather than separate interpretations of radiological and nuclear medical procedures. Daily review of this integrated material by the resident staff has facilitated a continuous critical appraisal and rapid accumulation of a pool of relevant experience. This has permitted us to quickly develop the criteria necessary to make accurate and significant nuclear medical diagnoses in pediatric patients.

References

1. CONWAY JJ: Radionuclide imaging of the central nervous system. *Radiol Clin North Am* 10: 291–312, 1972

Discussion

V. K. Chowdhary (Palmetto General Hospital, Miami, Fla.): In all of the cerebral flow study slides seen, none demonstrated a posterior flow study. What is the general opinion regarding posterior flow studies in children under the age of 10 or 12 years? Moreover, some of the slides seen showed that a dose of 15 mCi ^{99m}Tc was used for various age groups for brain scanning, e.g., ages 7, 9, and 10. Is it a standard practice to use 15 mCi or does it vary for a certain age group as such?

Dr. Gilday: We presently do all our cerebral radionuclide angiograms in the posterior position, because it is easier to inject the patients in this position and also at least 50% or more of the pathology is in the posterior half of the head in the pediatric age group. We use a much less flexed position than that for a routine posterior view. We use 210 μCi/kg of ^{99m}Tc-pertechnetate and occasionally of ^{99m}Tc-DTPA.

Jay S. Budin (Kaiser Permanente Medical Center, Sacramento, Calif.): The great majority of your scans for Meckel's diverticulum were negative. Have any of the negatives subsequently had a Meckel's demonstrated at laparotomy?

Dr. Gilday: No. All negative studies did not have a Meckel's diverticulum.

Ed. note: Not all Meckel's have gastric mucosa, either, so they may not exchange pertechnetate for chloride and not be positive on scan. These would not bleed or produce symptoms, either, fortunately.

Chapter 16

Radiobiology and Dosimetry

Eugene L. Saenger and James G. Kereiakes

t is widely accepted that procedures using any form of ionizing radiation in infants and children should follow the general concept that the potential benefit to be derived should exceed the implied risk. It is not necessary to shun such procedures blindly; similarly, when procedures are carried out in this age group, special attention must be given to the techniques which are used to conform to the principle of lowest practicable dose to achieve the desired clinical benefit. The physician, his technical staff, and equipment must have the skill and capability of performance to achieve this goal.

In this chapter, the recent reports dealing with low-level radiation effects will be reviewed briefly. In addition, some discussion of dosimetry and health physics procedures especially pertinent to pediatrics will be mentioned. The desirability of using certain newer radionuclides such as ^{99m}Tc and ^{123}I, which yield little or no particulate radiation and have short half-lives (significantly reducing tissue and organ doses), will be discussed. Unless there is a gross miscalculation in administering a radiopharmaceutical, no acute or clinically detectable radiation effects could be anticipated.

Radiobiological Considerations

Our prime consideration for purposes of pediatric nuclear medicine will be the possibility of late effects from low dose levels (of the order of 0.1–10 rem) and low dose rates (about 1 rad/hr or less).

This subject has been carefully reviewed by several expert committees representing international and national organizations over the past

3 years with the issuance of several reports and statements (1–3), such as those of ICRP, NCRP, BEIR, and UNSCEAR (See Box below). Also we have reviewed this subject as it relates to nuclear medicine twice recently, and these papers should be consulted for pertinent, older references to this general subject (4, 5). There are some significant differences in these reports which have some implications for the use of radiation in pediatrics and many major conclusions of agreement.

The most succinct statement following the issuance of the reports described above is that of the ICRP (6). It reaffirms its previous dose limits for workers and the general public which essentially correspond to those of the NCRP (See Table 16-1) and sees no cause for modifying them, either by making them stricter or relaxing them. The recommendations include the requirement that "all doses be kept as low as readily achievable, economic and social considerations being taken into account". The NCRP recommends that exposure be kept to the lowest practicable level needed. Both ICRP and NCRP exclude medical radiation from the dose limits of Table 16-1.

Somewhat in contrast to the above statement are the recommendations of the BEIR Committee. As paraphrased by Comar (8), its chairman, the BEIR Committee sought scientific assessments which need to be

---

Where to Order Reports:

International Commission on Radiological Protection:
ICRP Reports available from Pergamon Press, Inc., Maxwell House, Fairview Park, Elmsford, N.Y. 10523.

National Council on Radiation Protection and Measurements:
NCRP Reports available from NCRP Publications, P.O. Box 30175, Washington, D.C. 20014.

Advisory Committee on the Biological Effects of Ionizing Radiations:
BEIR Report available from Environmental Protection Agency, Rm. 635A, Waterside Mall East, 401 M Street, S.W., Washington, D.C. 20460.

United Nations Scientific Committee on the Effects of Atomic Radiation:
UNSCEAR Reports available from United Nations, Sales Section, New York, N.Y. 10017.

TABLE 16-1. Recommendations for Population Dose Limits of ICRP (*6*) and NCRP (*3*)

For individuals	0.5 rem in a year
Maximum permissible dose for adults exposed in the course of work	5 rems in a year

"sound", but also "they should be accepted as such by the general public". Thus a criterion of judgment of scientific data considerably at variance with those customarily used in many other circumstances pervades this report.

Lest this discussion seem to verge on the theological, it is necessary to understand how these various positions affect our thinking as pediatric nuclear medicine physicians. The difference comes in the daily application of *lowest practicable* levels of radiation vs. *lowest possible* levels. The latter term implies a definite, calculable risk to each radiation exposure which increases with dose—the linear non-threshold hypothesis. This assumption was used in the calculation of somatic risks throughout the BEIR Report. This relationship, similar to the Delaney amendment (*9*), which absolutely eliminates "carcinogens" in foods, seems attractive in principle, but it does restrict the thinking of physicians in regard to the utility of medical radiation procedures and urges for all radiation a zero release concept.

The data base for all of these reviews and estimates is essentially the same over the past few years. In regard to genetic effects of low-level radiation, for many years these were considered to be the most important as compared to somatic or developmental effects. More recent data, based on animal studies, have indicated that the genetic effects are probably less important than somatic effects. There are no applicable studies in human beings which show clearcut genetic effects, even at those exposure levels encountered during atomic bomb exposures (Ref. *1*, pp. 41–72).

Growth and development of the fetus and young individual can readily be affected by radiation. Present evidence indicates that the levels at which these occur can possibly be between 10 and 20 rads, but even alterations in behavior cannot be recognized until about 25 rads are given at some stages in prenatal life. The threshold for morphologic alterations in man following irradiation in prenatal life are less precisely known, but observations on the Japanese exposed to atomic bomb radiation place it between 50 and 25 rads to the mother (Ref. *1*, pp. 73–82).

Somatic effects of radiation have shown an increase in frequency in the two most important recent studies—those of the Japanese atomic bomb survivors and the British (Ref. *1*, pp. 83–91). The only important somatic consequence of low-dose radiation is that of cancer. Two of the best brief reviews of this subject are those of Miller (*10*) and Hutchinson

(11). The malignancies have been induced at relatively high doses and high dose rates. It is difficult to find appropriate populations exposed to low-dose and low-dose-rate radiation where the association between radiation and cancer can be considered to be assignable solely or chiefly to radiation; hence, the current risk estimates are an *interpolation* between zero dose and effect and the cancer mortality or incidence at high doses and dose rates. Risk estimates for several tumors are given in Table 16-2, which should be consulted for the very brief review which follows.

The most widely studied neoplasm is leukemia. All acute and chronic granulocytic forms are associated with radiation, but chronic lymphocytic leukemia is not. For the Japanese children exposed postnatally, when the relative or absolute risks are compared to those of the adults, the relative and absolute risks are increased by a factor of 1.7 over adults, indicating the increased susceptibility of children to radiation-induced cancer.

The effect of prenatal irradiation on leukemia and cancer induction in children is less clearly understood. In a widely reviewed series of papers, Stewart *(13–16)* and her associates have reported an increase in the frequency of pelvimetric or other obstetric irradiation in the mothers of children developing leukemia as compared to the frequency of maternal irradiation in the mothers of matched controls. These and other similar retrospective studies *(17)* are used to estimate leukemogenesis and cancerogenesis in those children exposed prenatally. Since the doses used ranged between 0.5 and 2 rads and the relative risk reported for leukemia was 1.5–1.6, these reports engendered great apprehension. No effort has been made to carry out appropriate prospective studies in medically irradiated mothers; that reported by Court Brown, Doll, and Hill *(18)* was not suitable for estimates of the relative risk at these exposure levels because of insufficient sample size and followup.

In 1970 Jablon and Kato *(19)* reported that in a group of pregnant Japanese mothers exposed to a mean dose of 50 rads no leukemias or other cancers were observed where 18.4 extra cancer deaths would have been expected using estimates based on the reports of Stewart and Kneale *(16)*. This prospective study raised a serious question as to the validity of these earlier retrospective investigations as had been predicted earlier *(20)*.

The conclusions of two recent reviews are of interest to the pediatric nuclear medicine physician in this evaluation. The BEIR Committee concluded that for the purpose of conservative overall risk evaluation, fetal or preconceptual radiation increases the risk of cancer in the child until 10 years of age but not thereafter. The UNSCEAR Committee *(2)* makes the following statement:

The effects of prenatal irradiation have been the subject of much research. A number of large surveys of children that were exposed to radiation for medical reasons before birth, and that must have received thereby doses of at most a few rads at high dose rate, indicate that prenatal irradiation is associated with a significant increase of the risk of malignancies in the first 10 years of life. The extent to which the increased risk of malignancies in the medically irradiated is due to radiation rather than to an association with the cause that prompted the irradiation must still be considered as open.

Cancer of the thyroid clearly shows an increase in incidence following many kinds of therapeutic irradiation in infancy and childhood, the relationships being similar whether studies are retrospective or prospective.

Similarly, relative risk estimates from the Japanese for all cancers except leukemia show that the age group 0–9 at exposure has an increased risk of 2.9, compared with 1.05–1.4 in the older age groups. Using the absolute risk model, the reverse impression is obtained with 1.2 deaths/ 10^6/year/rem for the age group 0–9 as compared with those of the older individuals, age 10–50+ at exposure, whose absolute risks range from 1.1 to 8.4 (21).

For these reasons, in pediatric nuclear medicine, the general principle that radiation exposures should be kept to the lowest *practicable* level rather than to the lowest *possible* level can be justified quite reasonably. Specifically, this precept means that, in each case, a priori, the expected benefit should have a clear opportunity to exceed the risk. More important, nuclear medicine procedures should not be used for screening purposes in children—the indications for each test should be clearly stated before the procedure is begun.

In regard to the use of nuclear medicine procedures in clinical research, we considered this matter at length several years ago (4). Without giving the details of the many considerations in this difficult area of medical judgment, the greatest problems relating to children are those of informed consent, particularly if control subjects are needed and if the research is not potentially of direct benefit to the proposed subjects (22). Nevertheless, the recommendations of reasonable dose limits for medical investigation as given in Table 16-3 may still be considered applicable.

Dosimetry

To present easily the dosimetry of common nuclear medicine procedures in pediatrics, Kereiakes, et al (23) have made measurements and calculations for standard children including newborn, 1-year, 5-year, 10-year, and 15-year-old children as compared with standard man. Body and organ weights are shown in Table 16-4.

The average absorbed doses to the total body and to specific organs for administered radionuclides can be calculated according to the MIRD schema of Loevinger and Berman (25):

$$\overline{D}(v \leftarrow r) = (\tilde{A}_r/m_v)\sum_i\Delta_i\phi_i(v \leftarrow r),$$

TABLE 16-2. Risk Estimates for Cancers in Children

Ref.	Study population*	Type of radiation	Mean follow-up (years)	Mean dose (rads)	Mean age at irradiation (years)	Relative risk (O/E)	RBE	% increase in relative risk/ rem	Absolute risk deaths or cases/10⁶/ year/rem	Remarks
						Leukemia (exposed under age of 10)				
1	A-bomb, H&N, 1945	G, N	25	69	5	19/2.93 = 6.5	1 5	8.0 5.1	2.6 1.6	All leukemia risks are for mortality
1	Thymus, x-ray, 1926–1957	X	18	65	0.5	6/0.96 = 6.2	1	8.1	3.0	
12	Head and neck irradiation, 1930–1960	X	20	65		0/3	1	—	—	
1	Tinea capitis, 1940–1949	X	15	30	?	4/0.9 = 4.4	1	11	3.4	
						Leukemia (exposed at age 10 or older)				
1	A-bomb, H&N, 1945	G, N	25	86	35	62/16.8 = 3.7	1 5	3.1 2.0	1.5 0.97	
						Leukemia (after fetal irradiation)				
1	Fetuses, England, 1943–1965	X	—	0.8	0	1.63	1	79	27	
1	Fetuses, U.S., 1947–1954	X	8	1	0	1.54	1	54	27	
1	Fetuses, A-bomb, H&N, 1945	G, N	10	50	0	0/0.15 = 0	1	0	0	

Thyroid cancer (childhood exposure)

	Study population	Type of radiation								Risks are for morbidity
1	Thymus, x-ray, 1926–1957	X	16	229	0	19/0.14 = 136	1	59	2.5	
1	A-bomb, H&N, 1945	G, N	24	143	5	6/1.60 = 3.75	1 / 5	1.9 / 1.2	2.6 / 1.6	

Bone cancer

| 1 | ^{224}Ra treated children. 1944–1945 | alpha | 21 | 1,103 | 10(1–20) | 35/.033 = 1,061 | 10 | 9.6 | 0.96 | |

All cancer except leukemia

1	A-bomb, H&N, 1945	G, N	25	69	5	6/2.1 = 2.9	1 / 5	2.7 / 1.7	1.2 / 0.75	
1	A-bomb, H&N, 1945	G, N	25	102	15	23/16.9 = 1.4	1 / 5	0.36 / 0.23	1.1 / 0.72	
1	A-bomb, H&N, 1945	G, N	25	86	35 (10+)	615/544 = 1.1	1 / 5	0.15 / 0.10	4.7 / 3.0	

* Columns: Study population—H refers to Hiroshima, N to Nagasaki; Type of radiation—G is gamma, N is neutron; for relative risk, RBE, % increase in relative risk, and absolute risk see BEIR Report, Chapter VII and Appendix B.

Note. For details, consult BEIR Report ("The Effects on Populations of Exposure to Low Levels of Ionizing Radiation," National Academy of Sciences, National Research Council. Washington, D.C., November, 1972) and UNSCEAR Report ("Ionizing Radiation: Levels and Effects," Vols. I and II, United Nations, New York, 1972). References are either to the published literature or to specific tables of BEIR.

TABLE 16-3. Suggested Limits for Doses for Radioactive Substances In Clinical Research (4)

Subject	Acceptable dose in 1 year (rems)	Acceptable total dose (rems)
Fetus	0.5	0.5
Newborn infant, child	5	5
Adult under 40	5	10
Adult over age 40	5	25–50

where $\bar{D}(v \leftarrow r)$ is the average dose in rads to volume v from radioactivity located in region r; $\tilde{A}_r$ is the cumulative activity in region r in $\mu Ci \cdot hr$; m is the mass of the target volume v in grams; Δ_i is the equilibrium dose constant in $gm \cdot rad/\mu Ci \cdot hr$; and $\phi_i(v \leftarrow r)$ is the fraction of the energy emitted by activity in region r, which is absorbed in volume v. ϕ_i depends on the gamma energy (MeV) and the source-target configuration.

When the target and the source are the same volume, then the above equation becomes

$$\bar{D}(v \leftarrow v) = (\tilde{A}_v/m_v)\sum_i \Delta_i \phi_i(v \leftarrow v),$$

where $\tilde{A}_v/m_v$ is the cumulative concentration in v.

The cumulative activity $\tilde{A}$ is related to activity A by the expression

$$\tilde{A} = \int_{t_1}^{t_2} A(t)dt$$

where $t_2 - t_1$ is the exposure time interval for which the absorbed dose is to be computed. The activity A(t) in an organ tissue is in general governed by these factors: the amount of administered activity, the site and rate of the radionuclide intake, the rate of biological uptake and removal, and the physical decay of the nuclide. In practice, measurements are made over the area or organ of interest and the effective half-life (T_e) is determined. The cumulative activity (for 1 μCi administered) can then be calculated for $\tilde{A}(\mu Ci \cdot hr) = 1 \mu Ci \times 1.44 \; T_e$ (hr).

Maximum thyroid uptake of iodine in the normal child is approached at about 24 hr. Mean uptakes of about 27% have been reported (26–29) and were used here for the 1-, 5-, 10-, and 15-year-old group (see Table 16-5). However, the uptakes of iodine by the thyroid of euthyroid infants during the first 2 weeks of life is high (30–34). Long-term data on the biologic half-life reported by a number of investigators reveal no significant variation with age (27, 35–37). A mean value of 68 days for thyroid biological half-life of iodine was used. A 3% uptake was assumed for pertechnetate in the thyroid. Cumulative activities for iodine radioisotopes and for ^{99m}Tc in the thyroid gland (for 1 μCi

TABLE 16-4. Body Weights and Organ Weights (gm) for Various Ages

Organ	Newborn	1 yr	5 yr	10 yr	15 yr	Standard man
Whole body	3,540	12,100	20,300	33,500	55,000	70,000
Brain	350	945	1,241	1,313	1,350	1,400
Heart	20	47	86	140	209	298
Intestines	146	398	550	820	1,350	1,700
Kidneys	23	72	112	187	247	300
Liver	136	333	591	918	1,289	1,700
Lungs	52	172	291	523	701	1,000
Pancreas	2.8	14	23	30	68	80
Spleen	9.4	31	54	101	138	150
Stomach	6.5	27	57	90	120	160
Thyroid	1.9 (1.5)*	2.5 (2.2)	6.1 (4.7)	8.7 (8.0)	15.8 (11.2)	20 (16)
Testes	0.67	1.5	1.7	2.0	18	28
Ovaries	0.29	1.0	2.0	3.5	6.5	8.5

* Thyroid weights in parentheses are from the recent data of Wellman, et al (24).

TABLE 16-5. Cumulative Activities for Iodine Radioisotopes and for $^{99m}Tc\ O_4^-$ in the Thyroid

Radio-nuclide	Effective half-life (days)	Newborn	Cumulative activity in μCi·hr* (1 μCi administered)				
			1 yr	5 yr	10 yr	15 yr	Standard man
^{123}I	0.55	13.3	5.1	5.1	5.1	5.1	5.1
^{125}I	31.9	772.0	297.0	297.0	297.0	297.0	297.0
^{131}I	7.2	174.0	67.2	67.2	67.2	67.2	67.2
^{132}I	0.1	2.4	0.9	0.9	0.9	0.9	0.9
^{99m}Tc	0.25	0.26	0.26	0.26	0.26	0.26	0.26

* Assumed uptake for iodine radioisotopes—70% (newborn) and 27% (1-, 5-, 10-, and 15-year-old and standard man); assumed uptake for pertechnetate—3%.

administered) are given in Table 16-5. Effective half-lives measured in our laboratory, and corresponding cumulative activities, $\tilde{A}$, for other radiopharmaceuticals are given in Table 16-6.

The nuclear parameter Δ_i, equilibrium dose constant, for the radionuclides was taken from the work of Dillman (*38, 39*). These equilibrium dose constants can be divided into penetrating and non-penetrating components as shown in Table 16-7. Particulate radiation and electromagnetic radiation of less than 11 keV are classed as non-penetrating. For the nonpenetrating radiation, since the absorbed fraction is 1, the absorbed dose due to the component is readily calculated. To use the penetrating equilibrium dose constants for absorbed dose calculations, an effective absorbed fraction for the target organ must be determined.

The absorbed fraction, ϕ_i, as a function of photon energy is available from MIRD (*39–41*). Absorbed fractions for gamma energies from 0.02 to 2.75 MeV are given for uniform distribution of activity in:

1. Ellipsoids of masses from 2 to 200 kg with principal axes of the ellipsoids in the ratio of 1/1.8/9.27 (for whole-body and large-organ calculations).
2. Small spheres (principal axes ratios of 1/1/1), thick ellipsoids (principal axes ratios of 1/0.67/1.33), and flat ellipsoids (principal axes ratios of 1/0.5/2.0) for masses of 0.3–6 kg (for organ calculations).

Ellett and Humes (*42*) have recently presented tables of absorbed fractions for small unit-density-absorbing volumes of 1–100 gm containing a uniformly distributed photon source. The data for small volumes are especially helpful for absorbed-dose calculations involving sizes of organs in children. The data for small volumes differ in one important aspect from absorbed fractions published earlier. It is assumed that the volume containing the activity is imbedded within a large scattering medium of the same composition.

Administered Activity versus Age

It is evident that the radionuclide activities administered to children in nuclear medicine procedures by no means follow a uniform pattern, particularly for the imaging procedures, where the statistics of photon detection per unit organ area become the important technical consideration. Webster (43) proposes the possible use of $[(x + 1)/(x + 7)]A$, for adjusting the activities normally administered to adults, where x is the child's age and A is the activity used in adults (see Fig. 16-1). This is a modification of Young's rule, $[x/(x + 12)]A$. However, the modification more closely approximates the criteria of equal activity per unit area of organ for most children's ages. Most internal organ weights maintain a reasonably constant fraction of whole-body weight with increasing age. The important exception is the brain, which tends to reach maximum weight by age 5 years. For this organ, Webster (43) indicates an administered activity schedule (^{99m}Tc-pertechnetate) of

$$\begin{matrix} >5 \text{ year } 0.1 \text{ mCi/lb} \\ <5 \text{ year } 0.2 \text{ mCi/lb} \end{matrix} \text{ (body weight)}$$

where the adult administered activity is 15 mCi (approximately 0.1 mCi/lb).

Radiation Doses from Radiopharmaceuticals in Children

Table 16-8 gives the thyroid dose resulting from the various radioiodine compounds and from [99m]Tc. The data also indicate the increased absorbed dose to be expected when the radionuclide is administered to newborn and children when compared with standard man. Whole-body and organ doses for other radiopharmaceuticals in children of various ages are given in Table 16-6. These data are for children administered radiopharmaceuticals in our laboratory after being referred for various diagnostic problems. Effective half-lives actually measured in these children were used for their dose estimates. Tables 16-9 and 16-10 were adapted from Ball and Wolf (44) except where indicated and show data for comparable radiopharmaceuticals and for other radiopharmaceuticals used for blood volume measurements and as scanning agents.

Certain radionuclides widely used in earlier years are now being replaced by newer ones which have shorter half-lives and decay other than by beta emission. Certainly ^{131}I administration is one of the greatest po-

TABLE 16-6 Measured Effective Half-Lives and Calculated Cumulative Activities and Doses for Various Radiopharmaceuticals in Children (23)

Age	Weight (kg)	Effective half-lives, T_e (days)		Cumulative activity $\bar{A}$ (μCi·hr) (1 μCi administered)		Dose (mrads/μCi administered)	
		$T_1 (C_1)^*$	$T_2 (C_2)^*$	Whole body	Organ	Whole body	Organ
				^{131}I-triolein			
3 mo	3.18	0.4 (98)	6.4 (0.02)	18.0		7.2	
2 yr	9.55	0.4 (98)	6.0 (0.02)	17.7		2.5	
				^{131}I-serum albumin			
2 yr	7.50	4.7		163.0		12.3	
				^{131}I-rose bengal			
5 yr	19.30	0.4 (0.90)	3.0 (0.10)	10.4	12.5	0.4	1.9 (liver)
13 yr	59.00	0.6 (0.80)	4.3 (0.20)	29.8	16.6	0.3	0.8 (liver)
				^{51}Cr-sodium chromate			
4 mo	8.18	15.0		519		1.8	
14 mo	12.60	20.0		692		1.7	
5 yr	20.00	20.0		692		1.2	
6 yr	13.62	19.4		672		1.6	
6 yr	18.60	16.5		571		0.8	
				^{59}Fe-ferrous citrate			
4 yr	19.00	26.0		900		49.3	
5 yr	20.00	38.0		1,315		70.3	
6 yr	13.62	31.0		1,072		78.0	
15 yr	55.00	39.0		1,350		32.0	

		C_1	C_2				
^{197}Hg-chlormerodrin							
3 yr	14.55	0.8 (0.82)	2.6 (0.18)	38.9	38.9	0.16	68.1 (kidney)
12 yr	47.28	0.9 (0.84)	2.6 (0.16)	40.6	40.6	0.07	39.0 (kidney)
^{75}Se-selenomethionine							
7 yr	24.50	0.8 (0.15)	23.3 (0.85)	689	689 (liver)	10.3	34.0 (liver)
					689 (muscle)	4.9 (pancreas)	8.7 (muscle)
^{47}Ca-calcium chloride							
7 yr	25.00	0.7 (0.94)	4.6 (0.06)	22.8	9.6 (bone)	2.8	4.5 (bone)
^{85}Sr-strontium nitrate							
4 yr	15.47	3.5 (0.38)	58.0 (0.62)	46.0	1,224 (bone)	16.3	68.3 (bone)
10 yr	32.70	1.3 (0.48)	44.0 (0.52)	21.6	792 (bone)	6.0	40.8 (bone)
11 yr	54.40	3.2 (0.20)	55.0 (0.80)	22.1	1,524 (bone)	9.2	62.5 (bone)
12 yr	40.00	1.4 (0.30)	53.0 (0.70)	14.5	1,283 (bone)	8.6	32.8 (bone)
12 yr	60.00	1.5 (0.65)	30.0 (0.35)	33.8	364 (bone)	2.5	14.0 (bone)

* C_1 and C_2 are fractional components of administered activity.

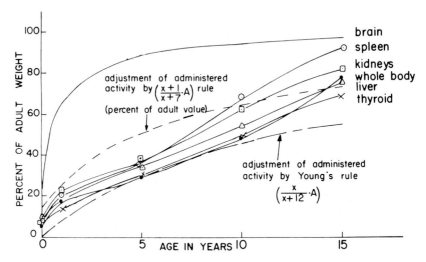

Fig. 16-1. Organ weights (percent of adult weight) as function of age in children (*43*).

TABLE 16-7. Total Equilibrium Dose Constants for Various Radiopharmaceuticals (*23*)

Radionuclide	Total equilibrium dose constants ($\sum\Delta_i$) gm·rad/μCi·hr	
	Nonpenetrating*	Penetrating*
Fluorine-18	0.5157	2.111
Chromium-51	0.0107	0.0612
Iron-52	0.4364	1.5640
Iron-55	0.0131	0.0000
Iron-59	0.2548	2.5083
Cobalt-57	0.0481	0.2590
Cobalt-58	0.0775	2.0935
Cobalt-60	0.2024	5.3321
Gallium-67	0.0776	0.3851
Selenium-75	0.0403	0.8185
Strontium-85	0.0195	1.1040
Strontium-87m	0.1421	0.6785
Technetium-99m	0.0362	0.2675
Indium-113m	0.2774	0.5601
Iodine-123	0.0602	0.3663
Iodine-125	0.0463	0.0861
Iodine-131	0.4135	0.8041
Cesium-129	0.0607	0.8362
Cesium-131	0.0168	0.0450
Xenon-133	0.2990	0.0896
Mercury-197	0.1579	0.1499
Mercury-203	0.2115	0.5066

*See text for discussion of absorbed fractions to be used with penetrating and non-penetrating radiation.

TABLE 16.8   Thyroid Doses in Children (rad/µCi Administered) (23)

Radionuclide mass number	Newborn* (1.5)	1 yr (2.2)	5 yr (4.7)	10 yr (8.0)	15 yr (11.2)	Standard man (16.0)
[123]I	0.160	0.109	0.051	0.03	0.021	0.015
[125]I	11.1	7.6	3.54	2.1	1.5	1.04
[131]I	16.0	10.9	5.1	3.0	2.1	1.5
[132]I	0.160	0.109	0.051	0.03	0.021	0.015
[99m]Tc	0.0068	0.0047	0.0023	0.0014	0.0010	0.0007

* Values in parentheses are thyroid weight (gm).

TABLE 16-9.   Radiation Dose (mrad/µCi Administered) from Radiopharmaceutical Scanning Agents*

Agent	Newborn	1 yr	5 yr	10 yr	15 yr	Standard man
Kidney scanning						
[203]Hg-chlormerodrin	2,480	800	500	317	242	200
[197]Hg-chlormerodrin	187	54	33	21	16	13
[99m]Tc-Fe complex*	9.3	3.3	2.3	1.3	1.1	1.0
^{99m}Tc-DTPA (bladder)†	4.9	1.8	1.2	0.8	0.6	0.5
Spleen scanning						
[51]Cr-red blood cells*	600	160	100	55	43	40
[99m]Tc-red blood cells*	20	6	3.5	2.3	1.6	1.3
Liver scanning						
[131]I-rose bengal*	10	4	2	1.3	1.1	1.0
^{131}I-MAA+	5	2	1.3	0.8	0.6	0.5
[198]Au-colloid*	380	160	93	67	44	33
[99m]Tc-sulfur colloid*	2.3	1.1	0.6	0.4	0.3	0.3
Brain scanning (dose to critical organs)						
[131]I-albumin (whole body)*	32	10	6	4	2.4	2
[203]Hg-chlormerodrin (kidney)*	2,480	800	500	317	242	200
[197]Hg-chlormerodrin (kidney)*	187	54	33	21	16	13
[99m]TcO4− gut*	1.6	0.4	0.3	0.2	0.13	0.1
thyroid blocked†	0.97	0.66	0.3	0.19	0.14	0.1
Lung scanning						
[131]I-macroaggregated albumin†	99.0	31.7	18.8	11.1	8.4	6.0
[99m]Tc-macroaggregated albumin‡	1.83	0.65	0.40	0.24	0.19	0.14
[99m]Tc-albumin microspheres‡	6.55	2.30	1.44	0.87	0.67	0.50
[131]I-macroaggregated albumin (thyroid)†	1,330.0	910.0	425.0	250.0	175.0	125.0

(Continued)

Agent	Newborn	1 yr	5 yr	10 yr	15 yr	Standard man
Heart scanning (dose to critical organs)						
[131]I-albumin						
whole body*	32.0	10.0	6.0	4.0	2.4	2.0
thyroid blocked†	373.0	254.0	119.0	70.0	49.0	35.0
[99m]Tc-albumin (whole body)*	0.20	0.07	0.04	0.03	0.023	0.02
[99m]TcO$_4^-$ (gut)*	1.6	0.4	0.3	0.2	0.13	0.1
Bone scanning (dose to critical organs)						
[99m]Tc-stannous diphosphonate or polyphosphate						
bladder-no void‖	6.27	2.06	1.19	0.76	0.58	0.49
bladder-void in 1 hr‖	0.90	0.29	0.17	0.11	0.09	0.07
skeleton‖	1.50	0.52	0.20	0.11	0.064	0.045

* Adapted from Ball and Wolf (44); † Ref. 4; ‡ Ref. 45; ‖ Ref. 46.

TABLE 16-10. Whole-Body Doses (mrads/μCi Administered) from Blood-Volume Measurements* (23)

Agent	Newborn	1 yr	5 yr	10 yr	15 yr	Standard man
[125]I-albumin	14.40	4.10	1.54	1.03	0.68	0.60
[131]I-albumin	32.0	10.0	6.0	4.0	2.4	2.0
[99m]Tc-albumin	0.20	0.07	0.04	0.03	0.023	0.02
[51]Cr-red blood cells	7.0	2.5	1.5	1.0	0.6	0.5
[99m]Tc-red blood cells	0.20	0.07	0.04	0.03	0.023	0.02

* Adapted from Ball and Wolf (44).

tential sources of high tissue dose, especially in very young children because of the beta radiation which is lacking in [125]I. This dose problem is best resolved through the use of ^{123}I since the physical characteristics of ^{125}I are suboptimal (47). Mercurial compounds also result in relatively high doses but are not now used widely because other more suitable radiopharmaceuticals are available for brain and kidney studies. It is evident that for many procedures, dose reduction can be achieved by using ^{99m}Tc-labeled compounds where possible. Strontium-85 results in relatively high doses to bone in children, but the development of diphosphonates and polyphosphates labeled with ^{99m}Tc for bone scanning have materially reduced dose contributions to growing bone and to marrow.

Health Physics

The term "health physics" usually is not used in reference to medical practice. The term originated in the necessary safety practices to limit radiation exposure for the nuclear weapon and energy programs. Perhaps it should be included under responsibilities of the physician and his colleague, the medical radiation physicist. Only a few suggestions for safe practice and optimal techniques peculiar to pediatric uses will be included here, primarily because many physicians and their staffs, who are thoroughly familiar with adults, lack experience in dealing with children.

The applications of "keeping the dose as low as practicable" requires some amplification. Nuclear medicine procedures are unreasonably long, both in an absolute sense and as compared with those of diagnostic x-ray. We still seem to be several decades (or eons) away from being able to obtain static organ visualization without motion of the patient. Hence, the radiation exposure received by the patient will represent a compromise between the amount of radiopharmaceutical needed and the sensitivity of the detector. It is important to realize that the dose of the radiopharmaceutical must be sufficient to provide excellent—not borderline— clinical information. If the images obtained are of poor quality, the administration is unjustified no matter how small the dose. If a nuclear medicine technique provides useful clinical information which can improve the management of the patient, the radiation dose should not become the limiting factor.

Bone scanning is an example of the change in our practice. The use of ^{85}Sr for bone studies in children was infrequent. The scans obtained were usually of poor quality, and the bone and marrow doses were relatively high. Strontium-85 bone scans were used, rather uncommonly, in patients with far advanced malignancy. It was not our practice to use this nuclide except in cases of suspected neoplasm. However, with the development of newer bone scanning agents such as ^{99m}Tc-diphosphonate, polyphosphate, and pyrophosphate, the scans are considerably better and begin, slightly, to approach x-rays in quality. There is also a marked reduction in dose to the patient. The effect of these newer pharmaceuticals is to permit wider use of bone scanning in children, chiefly because of the marked improvement in the clinical information obtained.

In a laboratory which does a reasonable volume of pediatric work (reasonable volume is defined by the physician in charge), radiopharmaceuticals should be obtained in precalibrated form and/or prepared and checked with a carefully calibrated laboratory dosimeter. "Quality control" procedures are necessary for each instrument used in the nuclear medicine laboratory. Appropriate calibration of rectilinear scanners is essential. The tendency for gamma cameras to produce artifacts or spurious images should be well known. The usual difficulty with these devices relates to the changing characteristics of the many photomultiplier tubes. Thus appropriate and frequent detector checks may be required and should be performed no less than once daily. All detecting equipment in daily use (well counters and probes) should be calibrated at least once both by background measurement and with appropriate standards.

Adequate immobilization can usually be done with restraints in newborns and infants. In the older child, it is frequently necessary to resort to sedation if the child is uncooperative (48). In cases of extremely ill children, we require the presence of a nurse or even a physician quite familiar with the patient's needs and disease during the entire procedure. The nuclear medicine technologist should not be expected to be capable of determining and fulfilling the special needs of these patients, particularly in the absence of a staff physician.

Summary

This brief review of radiobiology should indicate the reasonable limits of pediatric nuclear medicine. Together with the dosimetric information and the few caveats of laboratory procedure, the use of nuclear medicine as clinically indicated, maintaining doses as low as practicable, should be readily applied to pediatrics as specified in the other papers of this symposium.

Several years ago, in discussing benefits versus risks in nuclear medicine (49), the conscience guide (CG) was introduced as a unit, being defined as the referral rate to better qualified centers from a laboratory where expertise in a given test is lacking versus the total number of examinations done in that laboratory. When considering procedures in the pediatric age group, the physician is urged to use the CG to do only those procedures for which he and his staff have adequate equipment and experience. In this way, the best interests of the patient and physician can be insured.

Acknowledgment

This work was supported in part by Department of Health, Education and Welfare grants USPH 86-67-212 (FDA), TIGM 5 T01 GM 01247-13, and NIGMS 5 T02 RL 00074-07.

References

1. Advisory Committee on the Biological Effects of Ionizing Radiations, *The Effects on Populations of Exposure to Low Levels of Ionizing Radiation. BEIR*

Report. Washington, D.C., National Academy of Sciences-National Research Council, 1972

2. United Nations Scientific Committee on the Effects of Atomic Radiation, *Ionizing Radiation: Levels and Effects.* UNSCEAR Report of Official Records with Annexes, vols I and II. New York, United Nations, 1972

3. National Council on Radiation Protection and Measurements, *Basic Radiation Protection Criteria.* NCRP Report No. 39. Washington, D.C., National Council on Radiation Protection and Measurements, 1971

4. SAENGER EL, KEREIAKES JG: Safe tracer dose in medical investigation. In *Progress in Atomic Medicine: Recent Advances in Nuclear Medicine,* vol 3, Lawrence JH, ed, New York, Grune & Stratton, 1971

5. SAENGER EL: Some considerations of pediatric radiobiology in nuclear medicine. In *Pediatric Nuclear Medicine,* James AE, Wagner HN, Cooke RE, eds, Philadelphia, WB Saunders Co, 1974

6. International Commission on Radiological Protection: Reexamination of dose limits. *Lancet* 2: 1158, 1972

7. International Commission on Radiological Protection, *Recommendations of the International Commission on Radiological Protection.* ICRP Publication 9. New York, Pergamon Press, 1965

8. COMAR CL: An individual looks at the implications of the BEIR Report. *Pract Radiol* 1: 40–44, 1973

9. Delaney Amendment. *Food Additives,* Section 409 of Federal Food, Drug and Cosmetic Act, 1958

10. MILLER RW: Radiation induced cancer. *J Nat Cancer Inst* 49: 1221–1227, 1972

11. HUTCHINSON GB: Late neoplastic changes following medical irradiation. *Radiology* 105: 645–652, 1972

12. SAENGER EL, SILVERMAN FN, STERLING TD, et al: Neoplasia following therapeutic irradiation for benign conditions in childhood. *Radiology* 74: 889–904, 1960

13. STEWART A, WEBB J, GILES D, et al: Malignant disease in childhood and diagnostic irradiation in utero. *Lancet* 2: 447, 1956

14. STEWART A, WEBB J, HEWITT D: A survey of childhood malignancies. *Br Med J* 1: 1495–1508, 1958

15. STEWART A, KNEALE GW: Changes in the cancer risk associated with obstetric radiography. *Lancet* 1: 104–107, 1968

16. STEWART A, KNEALE GW: Radiation dose effects in relation to obstetric x-rays and childhood cancers. *Lancet* 1: 1185–1188, 1970

17. MACMAHON B: Prenatal x-ray exposure and childhood cancer. *J Natl Cancer Inst* 28: 1173–1191, 1962

18. COURT BROWN WM, DOLL R, HILL AB: The incidence of leukaemia following exposure to diagnostic radiation in utero. *Br Med J* 2: 1539–1545, 1960

19. JABLON S, KATO H: Childhood cancer in relation to prenatal exposure to atomic-bomb radiation. *Lancet* 2: 1000–1003, 1970

20. STERLING TD, SAENGER EL, PHAIR JJ: Radiation epidemiology. *Cancer* 15: 489–503, 1962

21. JABLON S, KATO H: *Radiation Dose and Mortality of A-Bomb Survivors 1950–1970.* JINH-ABCC Life Span Study. Report 6 (TR 10-71), Japanese Institute of Health 1971

22. U.S. Department of Health, Education, and Welfare, *The Institutional*

Guide to DHEW Policy on Protection of Human Subjects. DHEW Publication No. (NIH) 72-102. Washington, D.C., U.S. Government Printing Office, 1971

23. KEREIAKES JG, WELLMAN HN, SIMMONS G, et al: Radiopharmaceutical dosimetry in pediatrics. Semin Nucl Med 2: 316–327, 1972

24. WELLMAN H, KEREIAKES J, BRANSON B: Total and partial-body counting of children for radiopharmaceutical dosimetry data. In Medical Radionuclides: Radiation Dose and Effects. Cloutier RJ, Edwards CL, Snyder WS, eds, Symposium Series 20, CONF-691212, Oak Ridge, Tenn, USAEC, TID, 1970, pp 133–156

25. LOEVINGER R, BERMAN M: A schema for absorbed-dose calculations for biologically distributed radionuclides. MIRD Pamphlet No 1, J Nucl Med 9: Suppl No 1, 7–14, 1968

26. QUIMBY E, MCCUNE D: Uptake of radioactive iodine by the normal and disordered thyroid gland in children. Radiology 40: 201–204, 1947

27. GOODWIN J, MACGREGOR A, MILLER H, et al: The use of radioactive iodine in the assessment of thyroid function. Q J Med 20: 353–357, 1951

28. BERSON S, YALOW R: Quantitative aspects of iodine metabolism. The exchangeable organic iodine pool, and the rates of thyroidal secretion, peripheral degradation and fecal excretion of endogenously synthesized organically bound iodine. J Clin Invest 33: 1533–1552, 1954

29. OLIVER L. KOBLENBRENER R, FIELDS T, et al: Thyroid function studies in children. Normal values for thyroidal I^{131} uptake and PBI^{131} levels up to the age of 18. J Clin Endocrinol Metab 17: 61–75, 1957

30. KEARNS J, PHILIPSHORN H: Values for thyroid uptake of iodine-131 and protein-bound iodine in "normal" individuals from birth to twenty years. Q Bull Northwestern Univ Med Sch 36: 47–50, 1962

31. VAN MIDDLESWORTH L: Radioactive iodine uptake of normal newborn infants. Am J Dis Child 89: 439–442, 1954

32. OGBORN R, WAGGENER R, VANHOVE E: Radioactice iodine concentration in thyroid glands of newborn infants. Pediatrics 26: 771–776, 1960

33. FISHER D, ODDIE T, BURROUGHS J: Thyroidal radioiodine uptake rate measurements in infants. Am J Dis Child 103: 738–749, 1962

34. MARTIMER E, CORRIGAN K, CHARBENEAU H, et al: A study of the uptake of iodine-131 by the thyroid of premature infants. Pediatrics 17: 503–508, 1956

35. VANDILLA M, FULWYLER M: Radioiodine metabolism in children and adults after the ingestion of very small doses. Science 144: 178–179, 1964

36. ROSENBERG G: Biological half-life of I^{131} in thyroid of healthy males. J Clin Endocrinol 18: 516–521, 1958

37. BERNARD S, FISH B, ROYSTER R, et al: Human thyroid uptake and bodily elimination of I^{131} for the case of single and continual ingestion of bound iodine in resin-treated milk. Health Phys 9: 1307–1329, 1963

38. DILLMAN LT: Radionuclide decay schemes and nuclear parameters for use in radiation-dose estimation. MIRD Pamphlet No. 4, J Nucl Med 10: Suppl No 2, 7–32, 1969

39. DILLMAN LT: Radionuclide decay schemes and nuclear parameters for use in radiation-dose estimation. Part 2. MIRD Pamphlet No 6, J Nucl Med 11: Suppl No 4, 5–32, 1970

40. BROWNELL G, ELLETT W, REDDY A: Absorbed fractions for photon dosimetry. MIRD Pamphlet No 3, J Nucl Med 9: Suppl No 1, 27–39, 1968

41. SNYDER W, FORD M, WARNER G, et al: Estimates of absorbed fractions

for monoenergetic photon sources uniformly distributed in various organs of a heterogeneous phantom. MIRD Pamphlet No 5, *J Nucl Med* 10: Suppl No 3, 5–52, 1969

42. ELLETT W, HUMES R: Absorbed fractions for small volumes containing photon-emitting radioactivity. MIRD Pamphlet No 8, *J Nucl Med* 12: Suppl No 5, 25–32, 1971

43. WEBSTER E: Comparison of radiation dosage in pediatric nuclear medicine and diagnostic radiographic procedures. In *Pediatric Nuclear Medicine,* James AE, Wagner HN, Cooke RE, eds, Philadelphia, WB Saunders Co, 1974

44. BALL F, WOLF R: Zur Frage der Strahlen-Exposition bei der Anwendung von Radioisotopen im Kindesalter. *Monatsschr Kinderheilk* 115: 581–590, 1967

45. TAPLIN GV, MACDONALD NS: Radiochemistry of macroaggregated albumin and newer lung scanning agents. *Semin Nucl Med* 1: 132–152, 1971

46. SILBERSTEIN EB, SAENGER EL, TOFE AJ, et al: Imaging of bone metastases with ^{99m}Tc-Sn-EHDP (diphosphonate), ^{18}F and skeletal radiography. *Radiology* 107: 551–555, 1973

47. WELLMAN H, ANGER R: Radioiodine dosimetry and the use of radio-iodines other than ^{131}I in thyroid diagnosis. *Semin Nucl Med* 1: 357–378, 1971

48. CONWAY JJ: Considerations for the performance of radionuclide procedures in children. *Semin Nucl Med* 2: 305–315, 1972

49. SAENGER EL, STUMPE W: The future of radioisotopes in medicine: benefits vs. risks. In *Medical Radionuclides: Radiation Dose and Effects,* Cloutier RJ, Edwards CL, Snyder WS, eds, Symposium Series 20, CONF-691212, Oak Ridge, Tenn, USAEC, TID, 1970, pp 491–508.

Chapter **17**

New Instrumentation

Malcolm R. Powell and Victor Perez-Mendez

Several advances in radionuclide imaging instrumentation offer possibilities of significant improvement in pediatric nuclear medicine procedures. Coupled with new developments in radiopharmaceuticals, this new instrumentation may provide major opportunities for improved image quality, reduction of absorbed radiation dose, shortened examination time, and, possibly, reductions in the cost of nuclear medicine diagnostic procedures. Rather than attempting an encyclopedic coverage of new instrumentation developments, we will describe several approaches to improving nuclear medicine imaging, illustrating these comments for the most part with examples of work from the University of California at San Francisco. We will consider ways to improve principal parts of a gamma-imaging system: the collimator, the position sensing device, and the image storage apparatus.

Collimators

Considering first the collimator, it is apparent that we must strive to maximize efficiency with provision of spatial resolution as good as or better than the position sensing device we use. The collimators for a scintillation camera with $\frac{3}{16}$-in. resolution must have at least $\frac{3}{16}$-in. collimator resolution. Collimators are better developed within their design limitations than any other part of current nuclear medicine imaging systems. The length and width of channels in current collimators define angles of photon acceptance which provide much higher spatial resolution than we can use with presently available position sensing devices. This is done by using sufficiently thick septa that septal penetration by photons in other orientations is minimal for the photon energies of the collimator design. The convergent collimator for stationary imaging detectors actually allows improved image resolution by transmitting an enlarged image to the position sensing device, improving upon its intrinsic resolution. If a scintillation camera has $\frac{3}{16}$-in. intrinsic resolution, the convergent collimator can, by doubling the size of the image transmitted to the detector crystal, provide a $\frac{3}{32}$-in. effective resolution. At greater image magnification the effective resolution would be proportionately greater. The convergent collimator has already demonstrated its greatest utility in evaluation of small organs in pediatric studies.

A different approach to improving collimator function grew out of work in astronomy (1). Fresnel zone plate imaging can improve spatial resolution of radionuclide imaging systems while allowing increased detector sensitivity (2). The Fresnel zone plate imaging systems offer a third advantage: they collect holographic information which can be organized after collection to present a tomographic image at any selected level within the subject. Figure 17-1 shows a zone plate which was constructed for early studies by our group. It consists of a series of concentric lead rings which are mounted in plastic. The areas of each ring and each intervening space are equal throughout the entire zone plate. The photons emitted by the subject are shadowed by the Fresnel zone plate to form a hologram that is recorded by the position sensing detector. Figure 17-2 shows holograms of two and of four point sources. As the number of radiation-emitting points increases within the subject, the initial hologram soon loses any apparent meaningful relationship to the original subject. To make a meaningful image from the hologram of a complex subject, the holographic information must be re-assembled as a conventional image. This is accomplished by use of a spatially coherent light source (a laser) which projects light through the hologram transparency, causing diffraction of the transmitted light so that it can be transformed through telescopic optics which focus this light as a recognizable image of the original subject. By adjusting the focal distance of the lens system or telescope, a specific tomographic level within the subject may be brought into sharp focus. The re-assembled image is recorded on photographic film. Figure 17-3 shows an early image of a thyroid phantom derived from a hologram collected by a Fresnel lens system and conventional film as the position sensing detector (2). Although the image is crude, it demonstrates the great promise of the concept.

Several advantages of the Fresnel zone plate over a collimator have not been fully described in the foregoing discussion. As can be seen from the illustration of the zone plate, this "collimator" has a large sensitive area compared with a pinhole or multihole collimator. The high detection sensitivity of a zone plate collimator is to some extent reduced by the requirement that a greater amount of information must be recorded for a given level of resolution than with a conventional collimator for a sta-

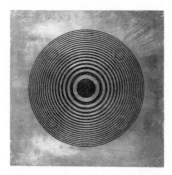

Fig. 17-1. Fresnel zone plate. Diameter of largest circle is 6 in.

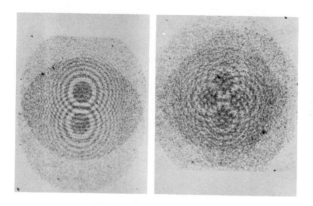

Fig. 17-2. Holograms of two point sources, left, and four point sources, right.

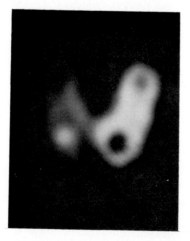

Fig. 17-3. Reconstructed image of thyroid phantom from hologram collected by Fresnel lens with conventional film as detector.

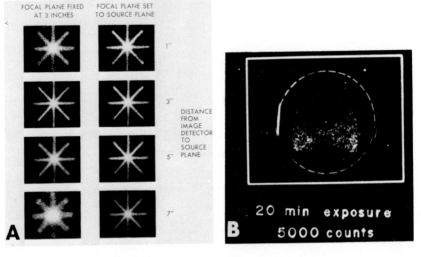

Fig. 17-4. (A) Resolution of positron scintillation camera. Source is ¼ × 12-in. rods filled with ⁶⁸Ge. (B) Positron camera picture of patient 20 min after 6,000 rads of 980-MeV alpha particle radiation to pituitary.

tionary imaging device. It appears that a significant improvement in the overall sensitivity can still be achieved. Additionally, a Fresnel system provides a high spatial resolution at a fabrication cost lower than that of current high-resolution multichannel collimators.

A different approach toward escaping the limitations of detector sensitivity imposed by multichannel collimators for stationary imaging detectors was proposed by Anger and has been available for many years (*3*). The positron detecting scintillation camera requires no collimator. Instead, two conventional camera detectors are used to detect annihilation photons in coincidence. The two detectors are referred to as the image detector (a conventional Anger scintillation camera detector) and the focal detector (a detector with a thicker crystal to provide increased efficiency for annihilation photons at 512 keV and containing fewer photomultiplier tubes). The patient is placed close to the image detector with the focal detector at a greater distance below the patient. When the two detectors record events in coincidence, both within the 512-keV energy window, the positron camera will sense and display the position of the positron annihilation. This can be accomplished since the annihilation photons travel at nearly 180 deg from one another and are displaced in opposite directions in the two detectors. The information from the focal detector is used to displace the position of the event recorded in the image detector a distance sufficient to display it as though it had been seen on a vertical above the positron annihilation. This so-called "dot-shifting" technique is susceptible to adjustments of electronic gain which will bring into focus various tomographic levels within the subject. Other levels will be present in the image but will be out of focus. Figure 17-4A shows the effect of focal plane adjustment at 1, 3, 5, and 7 in. as a pattern of radioactive rods is moved up and down below the image detector or as the rods are fixed in position while the focal plane adjustment is varied. The extreme sensitivity of the positron camera is well illustrated by Fig. 17-4B which demonstrates positron annihilation occurring in the region of the pituitary in a patient who had just received 980-MeV alpha particle irradiation of the pituitary at the Lawrence Berkeley Laboratory. The fanlike appearance of activation within the patient's head (which is not unlike the appearance of a radiation warning insignia) describes the entry and exit paths of the alpha particle beams which centered on the pituitary during rotational therapy.

Although the positron camera is little used in clinical nuclear medicine at the present time, it might be re-examined for pediatric applications. Absence of a collimator permits high sensitivity and high spatial resolution images can be achieved with smaller doses of radiopharmaceuticals.

Position-Sensing Detectors

Turning now to developments that might improve the function of our position-sensing detectors, several widely varied approaches offer promise. Although significant improvements continue to be made in the function of devices using the Anger principle of localization of a scintillation in a disk of sodium iodide, the use of other detector materials has been approached in a wide variety of ways. The primary problem is to produce a position-sensing transducer which can convert the energy of a gamma photon to an electrical pulse susceptible to recording by any of a number of devices, or display it as a flash of light on an oscilloscope. One new transducer that is still in the very early stages of development uses fiberoptics (4). These fiberoptics consist of very fine glass tubes which have a highly refractive outer layer surrounding an inner layer with a lower index of refraction. A phosphor can be deposited centrally within each glass fiber. Any ionization within the phosphor will cause light emission which is transmitted along the fiber to its terminus. Individual fibers can be made as small as 250 microns in diameter and assembled into parallel fiber transducers. The efficiency of the transducers is dependent simply on fiber length. There are no major handicaps toward developing detectors several centimeters thick. A light-sensing device such as an image intensifier tube would then be used to detect the image transmitted by the fibers. The advantages of a fiberoptic system would be high sensitivity and resolution but there would be no direct pulse-height spectrometry.

Another interesting approach to detector improvement is represented by the gas-filled chamber. We are currently interested in the development of pressurized multiwire proportional chambers (MWPC) for radionuclide imaging (5). These chambers provide high spatial resolution, uniform response, and large detector size at a relatively low cost. The major limitation of the pressurized MWPC at the present time is its decreased efficiency as photon energies increase. The MWPC contains three wire grids. The center grid is at a high positive potential and the two outer grids are near ground potential. The front window is made of Mylar or thin aluminum to minimize photon absorption. If the chamber is pressurized, the thin window is reinforced by a collimator built as an integral part of the chamber. Pressurization would be necessary to have useful efficiency for energies as high as 140 keV. The wire grids determine the position of photons which are absorbed within the chamber. As a photon passes through a collimator hole to enter the front window of the cham-

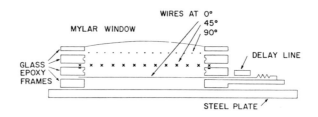

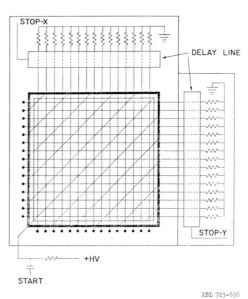

XBL 723-638

Fig. 17-5. Construction details of pressurized multiwire proportional chamber.

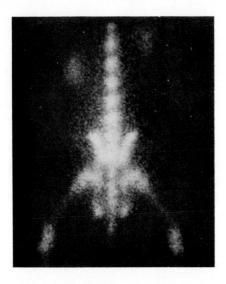

Fig. 17-6.   Bone image of animal taken with proportional chamber.

ber, it interacts with the xenon gas which fills the chamber. After photo-electric absorption the photoelectron drifts to the central grid because of the higher positive potential of that grid. Near the center grid, avalanche ionization occurs proportional to the energy of the original photoelectron. The avalanche induces "image pulses" in each of the two outer grids which are oriented at 90 deg so that their wires carry x and y position information to capacitatively coupled delay lines in close proximity to the grid wires but outside the margins of the chamber. Details of the structure of the chamber are shown in Fig. 17-5. The delay-line simply consists of a helical winding of wire around a central core with metal bars which form a distributive capacity for the coil (6). When a pulse is induced at one point on the delay line, it travels down the helical coil of wire to the end of the delay line with the travel time proportional to the distance travelled. The x and y coordinates are read out from the delay lines, and the central grid pulse is used for setting an appropriate energy window. Then digitized x and y signals may be recorded directly by a digital data processing system or may be displayed on an oscilloscope for photography. We are working on chambers which will be pressurized at approximately 5 atm and will have at least a 7% efficiency for 140-keV photons. Figure 17-6 illustrates an animal study conducted with such a chamber. The high resolution of the bone structure is apparent and would provide an excellent radionuclide imaging device for pediatric nuclear medicine, particularly if detection efficiency can be raised enough to compete with current devices. This may be possible by construction of larger MWPC detectors and by use of multiple detector heads on a single patient study to avoid time lost during position changes. MWPC detectors are much less expensive to construct than other currently available gamma detecting cameras.

Other approaches towards increasing the size of the field of view available with the current Anger scintillation camera include the divergent collimator and use of a 16-in. crystal, 37-photomultiplier tube camera. Both of these approaches have limitations. The divergent collimator will necessarily result in some loss of spatial resolution. The large-crystal Anger camera is an exceedingly complex device with resulting major increase in cost, and it has all the limitations of resolution and uniformity of response inherent in this instrument.

Another intriguing approach towards improving the performance of position-sensing detectors lies in developing better combinations of available technologies. Such an approach might involve using the Fresnel lens concept with a pressurized MWPC detector to obtain increased sensitivity and take advantage of the high spatial resolution and uniformity inherent in this detector. Another approach might be to use the MWPC detector as a positron annihilation radiation detector. This would require conversion of the 512-keV annihilation photons to electrons by use of thin lead sheet convertors placed in close proximity to the cathode wire planes of the chamber. Detector efficiency could be further increased by stacking several such detectors which would use a single readout device. Both approaches are under current investigation in our laboratory.

Other recent approaches towards improving the position sensing device have included the construction of a liquid xenon detector (7) and several approaches towards the development of a solid-state detector. Both types of detector are still fraught with many difficulties. The liquid xenon device has problems with impurities that develop in the liquid xenon with use, and this detector also requires elaborate innovations in design so that the liquid xenon can be maintained at cryogenic temperatures. The solid-state devices involve similar technologic problems since development of semiconductor crystals is quite expensive when their size increases beyond those currently available. Early attempts with high-purity germanium detectors offer some promise of a high-resolution, high-sensitivity device with the extremely high photon energy resolution that is available with these devices. Whether this energy resolution with virtual elimination of radiation energies outside the precise photopeak energy will prove to offer advantages sufficient to justify the expense of construction of a germanium detector remains to be seen from evaluation of test systems.

Image Storage Apparatus

The third general area where a radionuclide imaging device may be improved is in the data processing after x- and y-position coordinates are furnished by the detector. One must be impressed by the wide variety of digital and analog signal processing devices and a similar plethora of photographic devices which are offered in the market place. Unfortunately, the ratio between price of some of these devices and their frequency of clinical use seems to be quite an exponential function. Rather than trying to enumerate all the approaches which have been taken in the general area of image presentation and analysis, our comments will be restricted to mention of several of the principal problems confronting us in image processing and analysis with a description of an interesting approach to their solution.

Most forms of image storage and manipulation require that the stored information be in digital form. When the image is retrieved and displayed, the digital storage matrix appears in the display as a checkerboard array superimposed upon the original image unless the digital matrix is so large that its individual elements are not visible in the display. Unless these images are stored in at least a 256×256 matrix size, and preferably 512×512 or larger, the image on playback has a visible matrix pattern which seriously interferes with the definition of the margins of lesions seen within solid organs where there are fewer counts within the target lesion than its surroundings (i.e., "cold targets"). Unfortunately, the use of a large storage matrix involves considerable expense for computer memory. Similarly, fast dynamic studies can be stored with minimal loss of time between frames within a computer memory, but this requires a large memory even for the lower spatial resolution that is required in most dynamic studies. If a small computer memory is repetitively transferred to disk or tape storage, a significant loss of data occurs during the deadtime required for each data transfer. An interesting solution to these problems has been proposed by Williams who used a Hughes image storage tube as a high-resolution matrix for nuclear medicine imaging storage (8). In a $1,024 \times 1,024$ matrix configuration this tube offers storage of up to 100 counts per location at low instrumentation costs and with only the minor disadvantage that there is some data loss during transfer from the initial storage on the tube matrix to a magnetic disk. Subsequent to that initial storage, no further data loss occurs since data analysis is performed from the magnetic disk or an image is refreshed on a display oscilloscope. This new image processing device can obtain a $1,024 \times 1,024$ high-resolution static image or can accumulate sixteen 256×256 or sixty-four 128×128 rapid sequence frames with insignificant data loss as storage is changed from one area to the next on the storage tube matrix. This device also will allow numerical analysis to be made within regions of interest and instantaneous playback of all stored data despite the actual study time. It is an excellent example of what can be accomplished in approaching the multiple problems (image storage and analysis plus numerical data analysis with rapid random access to stored data) that are encountered in clinical nuclear medicine.

Summary

A rather wide variety of approaches are available toward improving pediatric nuclear medicine imaging. Hopefully, some that have been described in this brief paper and many other combinations will become available in useful commercial instrumentation. We think that we then will more closely approach the ideal situation where maximum use is made of the available gamma photons to obtain improved images with further decrease of patient radiation exposure.

References

1. YOUNG NO: A reticule camera. *Sky and Telescope* 25: 8–9, 1963

2. BARRETT HH: Fresnel zone plate imaging in nuclear medicine. *J Nucl Med* 13: 382–385, 1972

3. ANGER HO: Positron camera. *IEEE Trans Nucl Sci NS* 13: 380–382, 1966

4. TRIPP M: Fiberoptics camera. Personal communication, 1972

5. KAUFMAN L, PEREZ-MENDEZ V, STOKER G: Performance of a pressurized xenon-filled multi-wire proportional chamber. *IEEE Trans Nucl Sci NS* 20: 426–428, 1973

6. GROVE R, KO I, LESKOVAR B et al: Phase compensated electromagnetic delay lines for wire chamber readout. *Nucl Instr and Methods* 99: 381–385, 1973

7. ZAKLAD H, DERENZO SE, MULLER RA, et al: A liquid xenon radioisotope camera. *IEEE Trans Nucl Sci NS* 19: 206–312, 1972

8. WILLIAMS G, KAUFMAN L, POWELL MR, et al: A 1,024 × 1,024 image storage system for the scintillation camera. *J Nucl Med* 14: 465–466, 1973

Discussion

Thomas F. Budinger (Donner Laboratory, Berkeley, Calif.): I wish to comment on a few topics which you mentioned in your comprehensive coverage of new detector systems: liquid xenon versus gaseous xenon multiwire chambers, Fresnel zone plate and other collimators.

The liquid xenon chamber is operating intermittently in the hands of Derenzo and Zaklad at the Lawrence Berkeley Laboratory. We have no concern that the cold conditions will affect the patient as I see no difficulties with the human engineering of this multiwire device which has resolution ten times that of the Anger camera, and an efficiency equivalent to that of sodium iodide.

In the limit of perfect statistics the Fresnel zone plate has definite advantages over the usual collimator, which has a transmission of only 10^{-4}–10^{-5}. However, we are far from the perfect statistics, and it is still very much an open question whether the Fresnel zone plate will give you any advantage over the conventional pinhole collimator. Further, the resolution achievable with this device deteriorates rapidly with energy increase, and the requirements of optical reconstruction make it cumbersome to use though we have done digital reconstruction.

With reference to the pinhole, I am sure you meant to include this collimator in your discussion of divergent collimation. I think it is particularly applicable to this meeting in that the pinhole allows one to image defects of kidneys and other organs in the very small infant. In fact, as the Johns Hopkins group has demonstrated for cardiac-flow studies, one can use the pinhole with reasonable doses of technetium to delineate cardiac abnormalities in very small infants during the neonatal period.

Editors' note: See Fig. 19-5 for an example of the use of a pinhole collimator in pediatric renal imaging.

Chapter 18

Computer Imaging Procedures

Thomas F. Budinger

During the past 8 years there has been a rapid increase in proponents for and skeptics of the use of computers in nuclear medicine. The subject of controversy is what clinical value can we derive from digitizing and manipulating scintillation events for various modes of displays of physiological function not readily available on a single analog system. Usually after years of experience and practice with medical techniques and instruments, courageous or disappointed clinicians pose questions of efficacy. However, it seems the computer in the nuclear medicine laboratory has received the challenge prematurely, perhaps because of the high cost, perhaps because the digital manipulation and capacity of the display system were inadequate, perhaps because the hoped-for results were not readily obtained, even by the researchers. Arguments seemingly against the idea of computers in nuclear medicine are in fact usually directed toward the inadequacy of digital technology to acquire, store, manipulate, and present Anger scintillation camera data in a fashion which gives a visual impact appropriate for the diagnosis and continuing care of the patient.

Photopeak events are discrete signals with analog x and y positions that can be readily digitized and sent to a digital computer which can execute an optional program or algorithm for manipulation and eventual display to the clinician. One can argue that one general-purpose small computer system can do everything many separate analog systems can do. One needs a multitude of separate analog systems to perform the functions of a single digital system, such as extraction and display of time-activity curves, background subtraction, motion compensation, and section scanning.

The questions we should ask are (A) do the digital systems do justice to the Anger scintillation camera output, and if the limitations of these systems are overcome, what computer-assisted techniques would the clinician like to perform, and (B) can these be conveniently executed on commercially available systems? The answer to the first part is that most digital systems lose 20–40% of the data during high-speed studies and almost all the systems do not digitize the image with sufficient spatial resolution to properly represent the inherent resolution of the scintillation camera. The answer to the second part of the question is the topic of this paper; however, most systems are so cumbersome to operate that processing data by digital computer might take twenty times longer than for similar processing by a specialized analog system (e.g., brain flow studies). Even if we are seduced into trying the digital computer in some nuclear medicine clinical studies, the tedium of performing these procedures will diminish our ardor unless we also simplify the technical complexities and shorten by factors of 2–10 the time required for data manipulation.

My presentation centers around the system and the studies we are using at Donner Laboratory, along with aspects of the use of digital systems in pediatric nuclear medicine. The object of this chapter is to show some techniques of transforming data from the Anger camera to give a display of physiological function to the clinician.

Instrumentation

Historical aspects. Over the past few years computers of 8–32K-core capacity with word sizes of 8–16 bits have evolved at university nuclear medicine research and clinical laboratories (1–11). These systems have been hybrid systems using either a 1,600-channel analyzer or a small computer for initial data acquisition and, in many cases, a larger computer remote from the nuclear medicine facility for manipulation and a printout of the processed image or other parameters such as effective blood flow. Commercial companies such as Digital Equipment, General Electric, Hewlett-Packard, Intertechnique, Medical Data Systems, Nuclear Data, Searle Radiographics, and others have put together complete systems for the acquisition, manipulation, and display of data from the Anger scintillation camera. These systems cost between 45 and 75 thousand dollars and are just recently finding daily widespread use in clinical nuclear medicine. We have been using a system which evolved through interaction with Hewlett-Packard engineers. This is now their system HP-5407A with some added software features that allow us to image from the Anger scintillation camera (128 × 128 matrix) and also the Anger whole-body scanner which in effect requires digitization of an image 64 × 384 (Fig. 18-1). The design had pediatric problems in mind, as one of the distinguishing features of this system is the spatial resolution

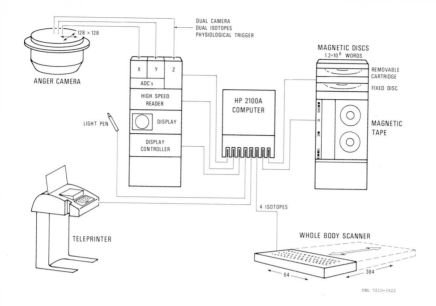

Fig. 18-1. Schematic of digital system configuration at Donner Laboratory. All parts of system except whole-body scanner interface are now commercially available.

and speed abilities. We considered the problem of doing flow studies in an infant with a heart rate of 180/min for establishing an upper limit for image framing rate (20/sec; 64 × 64). Below is a brief description of some of the important parameters of this system, which is a summary of a detailed report available elsewhere (*12*).

Analog-to-digital conversion (ADC). There are six important characteristics of the nuclear medicine ADC contained in the Hewlett-Packard system:

1. pulse pair resolution less than 3 μsec,
2. differential nonlinearity less than 1%,
3. 7-bit digitization in x and y (128 × 128),
4. ability to move the field of view,
5. ability to zoom,
6. capability of acquiring information from physiological triggers, different energies or isotopes, or an additional camera looking at the same patient from a different view.

The speed and spatial resolution requirements are vital to any quantitative nuclear medicine system, and it is in this respect that we felt most digital systems had serious limitations. During the routine 10 mCi ^{99m}Tc-pertechnetate or albumin cardiac study, the data rate of the photopeak events is 40 kHz during 2–3 sec of the study. With a deadtime of 20 μsec, the loss

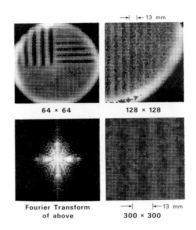

64 × 64   128 × 128

Fourier Transform   →| |←—13 mm
of above   300 × 300

Fig. 18-2. Illustration of inadequacy of 64 × 64 resolution digitalization. Right lower quadrant of 6.35-mm-wide bar pattern shown in left upper was digitized at 128 × 128 in right upper figure, and same pattern was digitized with resolution of 300 × 300 by using zoom control of ADC. Fourier transform shows power spectrum of entire bar pattern and is included to illustrate that small computer can do 64 × 64 Fourier transform in less than 1 min.

of data is 45%, and for 40 μsec, 62%. In fact, one can show that the maximum counting rate as the source isotope increases without limit is (deadtime)$^{-1}$, which for a 40-μsec system is 25 kHz. Slow systems not only limit statistics but give washout or flow curves which are distorted and must be corrected before they can be used for quantitative work. This is particularly important in pediatric cardiac flow studies. Correction of the observed counting rate to the true counting rate is impractical because the basic statistics cannot be improved

The clock time of the dual ADCs used in the Hewlett-Packard system is 200 MHz, and the pulse pair resolution for each ADC digitizing 7 bits is 3 μsec. Although most Anger scintillation cameras have a pulse pair resolution greater than 6 μsec (for the high performance cameras, about 12 μsec), other imaging devices such as multicrystal NaI(Tl), multiwire gas or liquid-filled xenon proportional chambers, or the pure germanium solid-state camera can provide data at rates of 300,000 Hz. In fact, the Anger scintillation camera can provide data with a pulse pair resolution of 3 μsec.

Spatial resolution of the digitized data should be at least 128 × 128 for static imaging using the modern gamma cameras. The argument for setting up a system with a resolution of 64 × 64 or 32 × 32 is that it is convenient for a particular 12-bit or 16-bit-word computer. As can be shown from the changes in the modulation transfer function, one needs more than 64 × 64 elements across a 10-in. crystal. Another argument, based on the uniform sampling theorem in a spatial domain, shows that more than 100 sampling points in each direction are required to faithfully represent the Anger camera data. Digitized resolution patterns show that a spatial resolution of 128 × 128 is required for a faithful reproduction of data available from the Anger scintillation camera (Fig. 18-2).

We incorporated the ability to zoom and the ability to move the field of view of our ADCs so that we could look with high resolution at small fields such as the upper chest of a premature infant or the midbody of a child. The emphasis here is to be able to digitize at high speeds using a frame size less than 128 × 128 by covering only that part of the crystal which is "seeing" the organ of concern. The zoom control involves no recalibration or complicated changes of the ADCs.

List mode versus frame or histogram mode. Framing speed is achieved in our system by inserting time markers every 10 msec during data accumulation. Thus in the list mode frames of 128 × 128 can be obtained at frame rates of 100/sec. A premature infant with a heart rate of 180 can benefit from a flow study if data are framed in 50-msec intervals. This figure is based on consideration of the wave shape of the time-activity curve over the precordium and the uniform sampling theorem in the time domain. List mode is an appropriate solution to the difficulties of moving buffer data into and out of core at these speeds. This mode allows simultaneous acquisition of data and gamma-ray energy or physiological information. Disk or drum data accumulation systems have the required speed to acquire data in the list mode, but tape systems are too slow for the cardiac flow studies we perform. Our system operates at 80 kHz in list mode and can operate at 300 kHz in histogram mode. In the latter mode the frame rate is limited to 10/sec on most systems. We have found that list mode not only gives the required time resolution but also gives the operator-clinician the option of choosing the intervals for framing of data. It should also be noted that in the histogram mode the capability of acquiring and storing 128 × 128 frame sizes is not present in most small computer systems since this requires 16K of core dedicated to this task. Our computer core is 12K.

The data are transferred to a raw data disk of 1.2 million words, which is adequate for most flow studies. A storage capacity less than a million words, however, will not suffice for nuclear medicine studies in list mode. If studies are done in histogram mode with a framing rate of 20/sec, it is highly likely that the accumulated frames of sparse data will exceed the disk capacity before the end of the cardiac study. After 14.6 sec the disk will be filled, and if the timing of the data acquisition commencement is not made at a proper moment after the injection, part of the study will be lost. Thus the storage capacity is an extremely important consideration in the argument for list mode versus histogram mode in high framing rate studies using a disk. The presence of a disk system gives a small computer the power and, in good part, the speed of program change that characterizes large computers.

System control. The computer system in a nuclear medicine laboratory can be as easy to operate as an Anger camera or rectilinear scanner. No special programming skills should be necessary. A child can run our system at Donner. The controls are teletype keys which have been labeled by a simple aluminum overlay. The study is started by depressing the key marked RUN and stopped by depressing PAUSE. Framing or regrouping the accumulated data is done by selecting a preset program initiated by depressing the key board program START or by entering framing parameters using the key CREATE.

Other aspects of the data manipulation and presentation require the intelligence of a technician, but not a computer specialist. These include:

FIELD UNIFORMITY CORRECTION: Floating point calculation which takes 11 sec to correct image based on flooded field.

FORMAT SELECTION: Display of any 4K block of the 16K (128 × 128) data; thus one can display 128 × 128 using four frames 32 × 128.

PATIENT READ AND WRITE: Transfer of frame data to and from magnetic tape for permanent storage.

KEYBOARD PROGRAM: Preprogram various phases of operation such as format, framing intervals, etc.

AREA-OF-INTEREST SELECTION: Up to 16 irregular areas of the image frame can be flagged and time-activity curves generated in less than 2 min for 160 frames or data points.

ARITHMETIC OPERATIONS: For both time functions and 4K frames one can add, subtract, multiply, and divide one frame or time function by another or by a scaler.

IMPULSE RESPONSE: Deconvolution of impulse response by application of Fourier convolution theorem to known input functions and output functions.

FRESNEL ZONE PLATE RECONSTRUCTION: Limited to 64 × 64.

WASHOUT IMAGE ROUTINE

MOTION IMAGE: Fourier transform of each element of a frame with respect to time to give frames of Fourier coefficients.

THREE-D RECONSTRUCTION FROM MULTIPLE TWO-DIMENSIONAL VIEWS

FRAME CREATION OR MASKING: Creation of a 64 × 64 image using the light pen alone or masking an image by setting all elements to zero outside the area-of-interest flagged data.

AUTOSCAN: Ability to scan through a sequence of frames automatically to play through a flow study or view an organ as it rotates in front of the Anger camera.

IMAGE ROTATE: Rotate images 90 deg by single key stroke.

PROJECTION OR ISOMETRIC DISPLAY

PROFILE DISPLAY

DISPLAY 64×64, 128×64, 256×64, 128×128.

CONTRAST ENHANCEMENT AND THRESHOLDING

SMOOTHING

COLOR PRESENTATION: By interposing Wratten filters between the P-31 phosphor screen and camera with Polaroid 180 film, color can be used to convey relationships of time or between isotopes.

MODE-OF-OPERATION CHANGE: System can be reconfigured to service a rectilinear scanner or other device in less than 60 sec.

OTHER OPERATIONS: Capability of operating on time functions or frames using BASIC, FORTRAN, or ALGOL.

Limitations. The basic limitation of this system is the inability to display 128×128 frames with more than six gray levels. Displays of 128×64 are done with mild scope flicker and a storage scope can be used to hold an image readout from disk, but this is not a satisfactory solution because of nonlinearities in image deterioration. Data can be displayed with no gray level on a storage scope such as the Tektronix 611 used by the Digital Equipment nuclear medicine system; however, the mapping algorithm used in that system suffers from a lack of a randomization routine.

Multiple camera operation during the same study is possible, but one cannot use the computer for more than one study at the same time. We have the ability to address the computer from multiple remote terminals and can timeshare on very slow operations, but most scanning procedures require a dedicated system to avoid data losses and facilitate completion of the data manipulation operations immediately after the study on one camera. Multiplexing is possible with large cores and has been done by Medical Data Systems; however, no reports on the logistics of multiple simultaneous studies on different patients have been published. A solution at present is to accumulate data on a portable read-write tape system equipped with ADCs, then at a convenient time take the tape to the computer for data processing.

With a disk operating system, tasks usually assigned to a large computer are easily accomplished. We do a 64×64 Fourier transform in less than 30 sec and plan to execute 15–19 variable compartment analysis programs in 15 min.

Techniques of Data Manipulation

Uniform field "normalization". Deviations of field uniformity up to 20% from the mean are not uncommon in scintillation cameras. The correction is important on both static (Fig. 18-3A) and flow studies (Fig. 18-3B).

Area-of-interest and time-activity curves. Selection of regions for de-

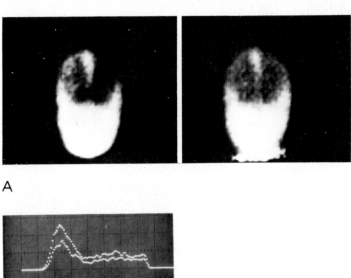

A

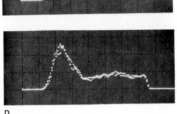

B

Fig. 18-3.   Importance of field normalization. (A) (Left) Before correction; (right) After correction. (B) False-positive brain blood-flow study corrected by normalization routine based on camera response to flooded field. (Top) Before correction; (bottom) After correction.

termining integral counts as a function of time can be performed readily for flow studies of heart and lungs (Fig. 18-4A), kidney, brain, and other organs such as parotid glands, thyroid, liver, and bone. Measurement of ejection fraction (13–15), cardiac output, right-to-left and left-to-right shunts (16, 17), and intracardiac transit times (1, 18) are easily effected using this system. No special reduced lighting or skills are necessary for the light-pen operation.

One can use the time-activity curves to aid in the visualization of phases of physiological activity such as the second and third phase of the renogram or end systole and end diastole (Fig. 18-4B). In the latter, data from periods of minimum activity and periods of maximum activity over the left ventricle are separated and summed to give a statistically strong image of end systole and end diastole. The minimum and maximum activity frames are found by differentiating the time-activity curve with respect to time and selecting the frames corresponding to zeroes in the resultant function.

Ejection volume can be calculated by this method using single-plane

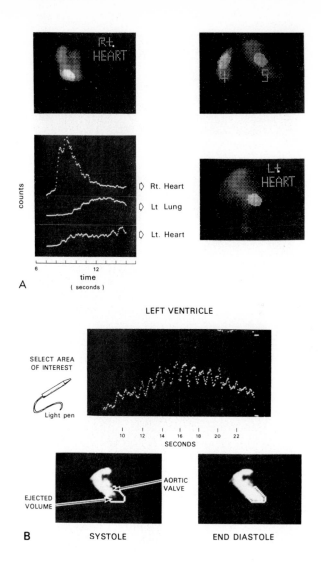

Fig. 18-4. **(A)** Heart and lung blood flow study. Left lower time-activity curves were generated from irregular areas flagged by light pen. Data are from frames accumulated at 20/sec using ^{99m}Tc-albumin, antecubital. **(B)** Example of retrospective gating where time-activity curve was generated at 50-msec intervals using area over left ventricle for count integration. Sum of frames at maximum activity gives image of end diastole and frames at minimum activity give end systole.

or biplane flow-study data obtained from cameras at 90 deg on the same study or different views on successive studies.

Arithmetic operations. Addition, subtraction, multiplication, and division of 160 point time-activity curves or 4,096 element frames by another time-activity curve or whole frame is accomplished by three key

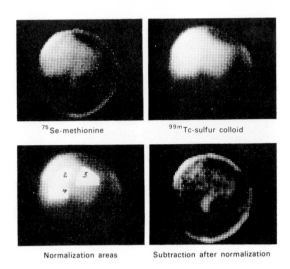

⁷⁵Se-methionine   ^{99m}Tc-sulfur colloid

Normalization areas   Subtraction after normalization

Fig. 18-5. Extraction of pancreas image by subtraction of ^{99m}Tc-sulfur colloid image from ⁷⁵Se-selenomethionine image.

strokes. The data for frames are accessed on disk automatically as part of the program, and these operations, including the transfer of the calculation result to a new frame, are accomplished in less than 1 sec. An example of image subtraction is shown for a pancreas study (Fig. 18-5). The activity over the liver for the ^{99m}Tc-sulfur colloid study is adjusted to that observed for the ^{75}Se-selenomethionine study by multiplying the respective frames by integers determined by the activity observed in selected liver regions in each study. Then the ^{99m}Tc-sulfur colloid normalized image is subtracted from the ^{75}Se-selenomethionine normalized image to give an image of the pancreas which supplements or clarifies, but does not supplant, the information in the original view.

Uses of Fourier transform programs. The Fourier transform can have an important place in nuclear medicine for effecting data analysis other than or in addition to image filtering. Both time domain and spatial domain one- and two-dimensional Fourier transform routines serve as the mathematical workhorse for the following procedures:

Spatial filtering. This potentially effective tool of imagery is not generally appropriate in nuclear medicine applications because of the character of nonadditive noise and change in transfer function of the object with distance from the collimator. This problem is the subject of intense investigation with only some special clinical applications likely in the near future (*12, 19–21*).

Fresnel hologram reconstruction. In work just completed with Macdonald, we have shown that the real space image can be reconstructed from the Fresnel zone plate image by applying a quadratic phase change to the digitized Fresnel hologram after which a complex two-dimensional Fourier transform is performed.

The efficacy of Fresnel zone plate image coding over pinhole imaging is questionable in nuclear medicine applications involving distributed sources. However, for studies which involve point source objects like the adrenals, this technique of reconstruction gives the curious clinician a means of exploring the usefulness of this new approach to collimation without necessitating acquisition of an optical bench and laser reconstruction apparatus. The digital technique requires 3 min with no film handling.

Motion image by display of Fourier coefficients. Periodic motion of an organ can be extracted from a study by display of the Fourier coefficients at frequencies corresponding to the periodic motion. Data from a cardiac-flow study with ^{99m}Tc-albumin are framed into 64 frames (4K) at 100-msec intervals. The time-domain Fourier transform is performed on time-domain vectors comprised of values from the same element in each successive frame. This is done 4,096 times; that is, independently for each time function vector representative of the same element in 64 frames. The result is a set of Fourier coefficients for each frame. Now the successive frames represent amplitude of the frequency at first and successive harmonics. The result is an image of motion with applications to heart, lungs, and liver. The 4,096 Fourier transforms consume 2 hr of computer time at present; however, with some hard-wired additions, this operation can be performed in less than 10 min.

Impulse response. Within the range of fluid volumes and injection speeds used in nuclear medicine, one can expect the organ of interest to respond linearly during the first few moments of a flow study. That is, the turnover function of the organ is invariant to the character of the input function. This turnover function is called the impulse response, and for linear systems where the observed input and output time-activity curves have good statistics, this function (which characterizes the frequency distribution of transit times) can be determined by application of the Fourier convolution theorem. The frequency distribution of an organ or system is independent of the shape of the input function, thus we have a method of describing the flow characteristics of normal and abnormal systems.

The system impulse response is the inverse Fourier transform of the system transfer function. The system transfer function is given by the quotient of the Fourier transform of the output function and the input function:

$$h(t) = \mathcal{F}^{-1}\{H(f)\} = \mathcal{F}^{-1}\left[\frac{\mathcal{F}\ (output)}{\mathcal{F}\ (input)}\right].$$

In practice this procedure is limited by poor statistics, inadequate definition of the input function, and the apparent nonlinear effects occasioned by recirculation (feedback). The program is a neat package which gives the response function as a time-activity curve after 4 min calculation (three Fourier transforms are involved), but has not been explored in clinical applications.

Washout or clearance images. If one assumes the disappearance of isotope from some organ region such as the myocardium or part of the lung is proportional to the fraction of isotope present at any time, i.e., $N(t) = N_0 e^{-\lambda t}$, the fractional rate constants λ for each region of an image can be estimated by least-squares fit of this simple relationship to data of successive images during a washout study. The product of λ and the amount present at $t = 0$ is the flow. This is the principle behind the washout or clearance images pioneered by MacIntyre (22) and Kaihara (23) and used successfully for lung studies (8, 24, 25) and myocardial flow studies after coronary injection of ^{133}Xe or ^{99m}Tc.

Poor statistics at the end of the washout study seriously bias the fit, and lead to erroneous values for λ, particularly if the usual linearized form $I(t) = I_0 e^{-\lambda t}$ is used. The proper function is:

$$\lambda = \frac{\sum A(t)}{\sum A(t)t}.$$

A check on the validity of the slope or rate image can be made by doing the computation using different time segments of the washout study.

Three-dimensional reconstruction. An approximation to the three-dimensional distribution of an isotope can be made from reconstruction techniques using multiple two-dimensional scintillation camera views. The objective is to delineate abnormal activity accumulation in regions of the body where surrounding normal activity seriously interferes with the diagnosis, such as posterior fossa tumors in children. The back projection technique similar to section scanning pioneered in nuclear medicine by Kuhl (6) is a rapid and relatively simple method of delineating tumors within the head. Other methods such as the simultaneous iterative reconstruction technique proposed for microscopy (26), the Fourier transform technique (27), the algebraic reconstruction technique (28), or the least-squares technique (29) are all in general equivalent and more sensitive than the simple back projection technique; however, they require 10–20 times more computer time. Our results in phantoms show the image contrast (tumor to background) of the iterative reconstruction techniques is as much as ten times that for the simple back projection technique. These procedures are available to nuclear medicine departments equipped with a computer and disk operating system. A patient study is shown in Fig. 18-6 in which 18 conjugate views were taken 6 hr after 8 mCi ^{99m}Tc-pertechnetate was injected in a 14-year-old girl with a suspected brain lesion (30).

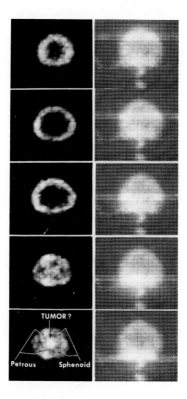

Fig. 18-6. Transverse section images calculated from multiple gamma camera views of 14-year-old patient's head 6 hr after injection of 8 mCi ^{99m}Tc-pertechnetate. Suspected craniopharyngioma.

Data Presentation

Contrast enhancement and background subtraction. Contrast enhancement and thresholding, or background cutoff, are two of the most important features of a digital, or for that matter analog, data storage system. The match of the two-dimensional data array displayed on a cathode-ray tube to the human eye has been a problem from the earliest days of nuclear medicine imaging (*31–33*). Detection of lesions is aided by changes in contrast and brightness of the display scope, but in some cases artifacts are enhanced. Control over the image presentation cannot always be obtained by simple integration of each dot on film using multiple f-stops as is usually done on the commercial scintillation cameras. In the situation where the differences in detected counting rate between a region of interest and the surrounding normal tissues is only 15%, some background subtraction or thresholding is necessary for visualizing the difference. The digital computer allows one to present the same study as multiple images using different threshold or cutoff levels.

Enhancement by spatial filtering and digital smoothing certainly gives images more appealing to the eye; however, investigators (*34*) have not found these techniques improve overall diagnostic accuracy. Results of image nonlinear restoration techniques such as adaptive filters (*19*) and histogram linearization procedures have not had clinical trials.

Techniques of contrast enhancement, and filtering by both smoothing and CRT defocusing, are illustrated (Fig. 18-7) for a lateral brain scintigram 1 hr after i.v. injection of ^{99m}Tc-pertechnetate. These well-known techniques are aids to the clinician who wishes to record an image which represents the optimal visual representation of his diagnostic impression. The dangers of enhancing artifacts by contrast enhancement of smoothed data are no greater than those experienced with other display techniques used with rectilinear scanners and scintillation cameras. The elective control of stored digital data can be obtained with special analog systems, but their cost is almost one-third that of an entire computer disk operating system.

Projections and profiles. The ability to show isometric projections and to display the profile of activity versus position gives the clinician or investigator a means of evaluating the statistical significance of suspected lesions or abnormalities (Fig. 18-8). The accumulation of ^{129}Cs in the myocardium can be made to appear dramatically great relative to the accumulation in contiguous lung and muscle by contrast enhancement; however, the true relative distribution is forced on the observer by the pseudoquantitative technique of viewing the isometric display (Fig. 18-8, lower right). This maneuver is a hard-wired algorithm available on most

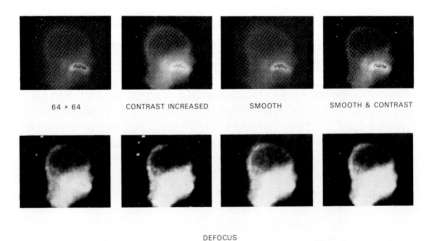

64 × 64   CONTRAST INCREASED   SMOOTH   SMOOTH & CONTRAST

DEFOCUS

Fig. 18-7. Manipulation of scintiphoto data. Example of methods of contrast enhancement and smoothing easily implemented by control of display module.

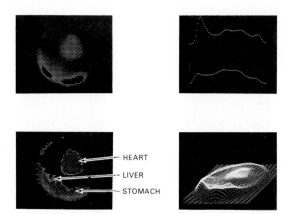

Fig. 18-8. Methods of displaying heart muscle accumulation of ^{129}Cs after intra-venous injection of 500 μCi. Profiles (upper right) give information on relative activity which cannot be obtained on conventional image (upper left). See text for explanation of lower figures.

nuclear medicine digital computer or analog display systems. Our system can execute rotation of the image by 90-deg increments, which facilitates looking "behind" the image. The time required to effect these maneuvers is 1 sec or almost as fast as a switch or key can be depressed.

Counts or activity levels of any magnitude can be delineated by adjusting a baseline and window width by analog controls on the display console. The picture elements having values lying within the window are intensified as illustrated in Fig. 18-8 (lower left). We have found only limited clinical advantage of this capability by following the contour of isotope movement through the kidneys.

Color. Color images have seven potentially useful applications in nuclear medicine. On a single scintiphoto, color gives the ability:

1. to give isocount or "gray level" delineation,
2. to represent different time intervals for a flow study (*12*),
3. to show respective spatial distribution of two isotopes,
4. to delineate relationships of transmission and emission studies on a single image,
5. to show relationships between ventilation or clearance and perfusion in the lung and heart studies (*25*),
6. to show relationship between static or anatomic image and the motion image by using color to represent each mode on the same print,
7. for facilitating stereoviewing using red and green images and red and green glasses.

We have found color very effective in delineating time relationships and in demonstrating the difference in uptake of two or three isotopes. Uses 6 and 7 are still research studies. Important relationships between right and left heart can be seen by using color to delineate time relationships. Other uses include radionuclide cisternography, cerebral angiography, and renography. The color images are obtained using red, blue, and green filters handplaced between the P-31 phosphor of the Hewlett-Packard scope and Polaroid 180 film mounted on a Tektronix CRT-camera adaptor.

Summary

The following clinically valuable adjuncts to nuclear medicine procedures are provided by a digital computer disk operating system:

Control of image data presentation including capability to use color, to correct for field nonuniformity, to enhance contrast, and to play-back study for reviewing flow or reflux.
Creation of time-activity curves from flow studies of brain, heart, thyroid, kidneys, lungs, and liver.
Quantitation of the counts or activity distribution.
Manipulation of data for the determination of physiologic parameters such as cerebral flow transit times, cardiac left-to-right and right-to-left shunts, liver function, heart function, and kidney function.

By having a state-of-the-art digital system at the technician's finger tips, you can provide your patient with the benefits of the above data manipulation and reduction techniques and, in addition, will be able to take advantage of three-dimensional reconstruction and motion extraction programs just now being implemented for small computers.

Acknowledgments

This work was supported by the U. S. Atomic Energy Commission. Assistance of Mary Lou Nohr, Marcy Wales, Grant Gullberg, and John Harpootlian is gratefully acknowledged.

References

1. ADAM WE, SCHENCK P, KAMPMANN H, et al: Investigation of cardiac dynamics using scintillation camera and computer. In *Medical Radioisotope Scintigraphy,* vol 2, Vienna, IAEA, 1969, pp 77–91

2. ASHBURN WL, MOSER KM, GUISAN M: Digital and analog processing of Anger camera data with a dedicated computer-controlled system. *J Nucl Med* 11: 680–688, 1970

3. BRILL AB, ERICKSON JJ, LINDAHL CD: Digital systems for data acquisition and storage. In *Quantitative Organ Visualization in Nuclear Medicine,* Kenny PJ, Smith EM, eds, Coral Gables, University of Miami Press, 1971 pp 339–379

4. BROWN DW: Digital computer analysis and display of the radionuclide scan. *J Nucl Med* 5: 802–806, 1964

5. COX JR, HILL RL: Design considerations for interfacing computers to gamma-ray cameras. In *Quantitative Organ Visualization in Nuclear Medicine,* Kenny PJ, Smith EM, eds, Coral Gables, University of Miami Press, 1971, pp 465–480

6. KUHL DE, EDWARDS RQ: Reorganizing data from transverse section scans of the brain using digital processing. *Radiology* 91: 975–983, 1968

7. LAUGHLIN JS, WEBER DA, BENUA RS, et al: Quantitative storage, analysis and display in digital scanning. In *Fundamental Problems in Scanning,* Gottschalk A, Beck R, eds, Springfield, C. C Thomas, 1968, pp 267–276

8. LOKEN MK, PONTO RA, BACH R, et al: Intravenous radioisotope angiography with computer processing of data. *Am J Roentgenol Radium Ther Nucl Med* 112: 682–690, 1971

9. PIZER SM, VETTER HG: Processing radioisotope scans. *J Nucl Med* 10: 150–154, 1969

10. POTCHEN EJ, BENTLEY R, GERTH W, et al: A means for the scintigraphic imaging of regional brain dynamics. Regional cerebral blood flow and regional cerebral blood volume. In *Medical Radioisotope Scintigraphy,* vol 2, Vienna, IAEA, 1969, pp 577–583

11. WAGNER HN, NATARAJAN TK, KNOWLES L, et al: Practical applications of the computer in radionuclide imaging, In *Medical Radioisotope Scintigraphy,* vol 1, Vienna, IAEA, 1973, pp 459–484

12. BUDINGER TF: Clinical and research quantitative nuclear medicine system. In *Medical Radioisotope Scintigraphy,* vol 1, Vienna, IAEA, 1973, pp 501–551

13. VAN DYKE D, ANGER HO, SULLIVAN RW, et al: Cardiac evaluation from radioisotope dynamics. *J Nucl Med* 13: 585–592, 1972

14. WEBER PM, DOS REMEDIOS LV, JASKO IA: Quantitative radioisotopic angiocardiography. *J Nucl Med* 13: 815–822, 1972

15. PARKER JA, SECKER-WALKER R, HILL R, et al: A new technique for the calculation of left ventricular ejection fraction. *J Nucl Med* 13: 649–651, 1972

16. MALTZ DL, TREVES S: Quantification of left-to-right shunts by radionuclide angiocardiography in children. *J Nucl Med* 13: 787–788, 1972

17. ALAZRAKI NP, ASHBURN WL, HAGAN A, et al: Detection of left-to-right cardiac shunts with the scintillation camera pulmonary dilution curve. *J Nucl Med* 13: 142–147, 1972

18. ISHII Y, MACINTYRE WJ: Measurement of heart chamber volumes by analysis of dilution curves simultaneously recorded by scintillation camera. *Circulation* 44: 37–46, 1971

19. KIRCH DL, BROWN DW: Recent advances in digital processing static and dynamic scintigraphic data. In *Sharing of Computer Programs and Technology in Nuclear Medicine,* Oak Ridge, Tenn USAEC, CONF-720430, 1972, pp 27–54

20. IINUMA TA: Image enhancement by the iterative approximation method. In *Quantitative Organ Visualization in Nuclear Medicine,* Kenny PJ, Smith EM, eds, Coral Gables, University of Miami Press, 1971, pp 549–562

21. METZ CE: A mathematical investigation of radioisotope scan image processing. PhD thesis. Univ of Penn, 1970

22. MACINTYRE WJ, INKLEY SR, ROTH E, et al: Spatial recording of disappearance constants of ^{133}xenon washout from the lung. *J Lab Clin Med* 76: 701–712, 1970

23. KAIHARA S, NATARAJAN TK, WAGNER HN, et al: Construction of a functional image from regional rate constants, *J Nucl Med* 10: 347–348, 1969

24. NATARAJAN TK, WAGNER HN: "Functional imaging" of regional ventilation and perfusion of the lungs. *J Nucl Med* 13: 456, 1972

25. BURDINE JA, ALAGARSAMY V, RYDER LA, et al: Quantitative functional images of regional ventilation and perfusion. *J Nucl Med* 13: 933–938, 1972

26. GILBERT P: Iterative methods for the reconstruction of a three-dimensional object from projections. *J Theor Biol* 36: 105–117, 1972

27. KLUG A, CROWTHER RA: Three-dimensional image reconstruction from the viewpoint of information theory. *Nature* 238: 435–440, 1972

28. GORDON R, BENDER R, HERMAN GT: Algebraic reconstruction techniques (ART) for three-dimensional electron microscopy and x-ray photography. *J Theor Biol* 29: 471–481, 1970

29. GOITEIN M: Three-dimensional density reconstruction from a series of two-dimensional projections, *Nucl Instr Methods* 101: 509–518, 1971

30. BUDINGER TF, GULLBERG GT: *Three-Dimensional Reconstruction in Nuclear Medicine by Iterative Least Squares and Fourier Transform Techniques.* Lawrence Berkeley Laboratory Report No 2146, 1974

31. BENDER MA, BLAU M: Data presentation in radioisotope scanning: contrast enhancement. In *Progress in Medical Radioisotope Scanning,* Kniseley RM, Andrews GA, Harris CC, eds, Oak Ridge, Tenn, USAEC, 1962, pp 105–112

32. HARBERT JC, ASHBURN WL: Selection of Polaroid film for scintiphotography. *J Nucl Med* 10: 127–132, 1969

33. CARLSON JC: Matching gray scale display programs to various film types. In *Sharing of Computer Programs and Technology in Nuclear Medicine,* Oak Ridge, Tenn, USAEC, CONF-720430, 1972, pp 207–213

34. KUHL DE, SANDERS TD, EDWARDS RQ, et al: Failure to improve observer performance with scan smoothing. *J Nucl Med* 13: 752–757, 1973

35. BUDINGER TF, YANO Y: Myocardial function evaluation by uptake of ^{129}Cs. *J Nucl Med* 13: 417–418, 1972

Chapter 19

New Horizons

Hirsch Handmaker

In view of the preceding chapters, the reader can appreciate the rapid changes that have been occurring in the clinical practice of pediatric nuclear medicine. Nonetheless, most of these procedures are actually routine in hospitals throughout the world, and with few exceptions, can be done on 24-hr notice wherever a gamma camera, scanner, and well detector are found. Only preplanned studies, sufficient hands for holding and positioning, and occasionally, recording devices for replay and analysis, are required.

What lies ahead? To hazard a guess seems difficult. Instead, the author choses to look at what is already being investigated for clinical utility and suggest some exciting new areas that may offer promise to the pediatrician and nuclear medicine specialist. Just as the "Meckelogram" provides a fast, safe method for identifying ectopic gastric mucosa producing unexplained gastrointestinal bleeding (1–3) (Fig. 19-1), a variety of enig-

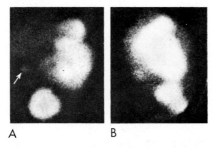

A   B

Fig. 19-1. 15-month-old boy with intermittent gastrointestinal bleeding. (A) Anterior abdominal scintiphoto 2 hr after intravenous injection of 1 mCi of ^{99m}Tc-pertechnetate demonstrates increased activity (arrow) in ectopic gastric mucosa between normal gastric, small bowel, and bladder activity. (B) Lateral view shows relatively posterior location of gastric tissue (surgically confirmed).

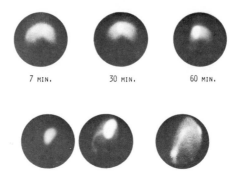

Fig. 19-2. Hepatobiliary scintiphoto study in dog using ^{99m}Tc-mercaptocarboxylate. Lower row are high-resolution images of gallbladder and common bile duct. (Courtesy of H. S. Winchell.)

matic pediatric problems may be solved in the near future using nuclear medicine procedures.

Hepatobiliary Evaluation

As mentioned in Chapter 7, there have been disappointing clinical results in differentiating neonatal hepatitis from biliary atresia. Recent reports of high-resolution, lower radiation exposure materials (*4, 5*) such as ^{99m}Tc-mercaptocarboxylate, appear encouraging in this problem (Fig. 19-2). The ability to better delineate the biliary tree in infants would be of great value. Likewise, this agent appears to be a single compartment tracer (that is, one that will leave the blood as a uniform function of liver cell integrity), making it an ideal means of evaluating liver function even in the presence of jaundice (Fig. 19-3). It would provide visual information of excretion patterns, like ^{131}I-rose bengal, with superior anatomical resolution.

Renal Imaging

As outlined by Conway in Chapter 9, certain techniques for evaluating children have been developed that not only add considerable information to the renal workup, but do so at a reduced radiation exposure. Our modification of various techniques (i.v. injection of a GFR agent ^{99m}Tc-Sn-DTPA) also eliminates the need for catheterization in evaluating children with vesicoureteral reflux (Fig. 19-4) (*6*).

Similarly, a new agent for renal cortical imaging, ^{99m}Tc-dimercaptosuccinic acid (DMSA) (*7*), appears to offer excellent capability for the evaluation of renal size and cortical integrity. Many authors feel that there is value in establishing the changes of chronic pyelonephritis as early as

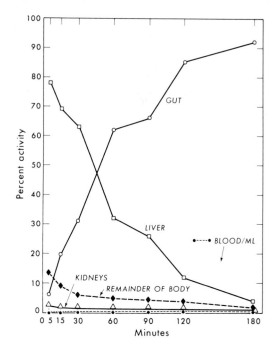

Fig. 19-3. Clearance curves for hepatobiliary agent in Fig. 19-2. (Courtesy of H. S. Winchell.)

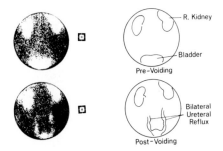

Fig. 19-4. Pre- and postvoiding scintiphotos 1 hr after the intravenous injection of ^{99m}Tc-Sn-DTPA demonstrating bilateral ureteral reflux in teenage boy.

possible (8, 9). Using a pinhole collimator and ^{99m}Tc-DMSA, we have evaluated renal cortical detail in a variety of patients (10), including the patient seen in Fig. 19-5, a boy with bilateral chronic pyelonephritis secondary to reflux. The severe cortical changes were not well appreciated on routine excretory urograms.

Yet another application in nuclear medicine in pediatric urologic problems may be in the atraumatic quantitation of differential renal cortical function and residual bladder volume and bladder mechanics (11).

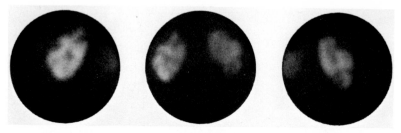

Fig. 19-5. Posterior static renal scintiphotos 2 hr after intravenous injection of ^{99m}Tc-DMSA. Patient is 15-year-old boy with bilateral reimplanted ureters in sigmoid because of bladder exstrophy. Marked deformity and scarring of cortex characteristic in pyelonephritis is clearly demonstrated. Left is left posterior oblique; right is right posterior oblique. Oblique scintiphotos made with pinhole collimator. Middle is posterior view.

Not only are these procedures of high diagnostic yield and atraumatic in nature, but most of them offer reduction in radiation exposure to below that of standard urographic techniques.

Cardiopulmonary Studies

The preceding discussion, like those of Kriss and Ashburn, emphasizes that valuable physiological information can be routinely obtained in addition to anatomic data. This perhaps is the real challenge and role of nuclear medicine and the horizon for its application in pediatrics. The possibilities inherent in very short half-life radionuclides are intriguing, particularly in pediatrics. Krypton-81m gas ($T_{1/2} = 13$ sec) can be ob-

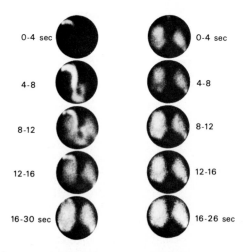

Fig. 19-6. Perfusion (left) and ventilation (right) study of right heart and lungs following intravenous injection of ^{81m}Kr. (Reprinted from Ref *12.*)

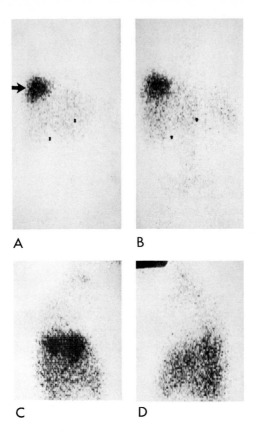

A   B

C   D

Fig. 19-7. Three-year-old boy with granulomatous disease of childhood, presenting with spiking low-grade fevers and vague abdominal discomfort for 1 week before admission. Scan performed after intravenous injection of ^{67}Ga-citrate shows scanty normal uptake of material by liver and axial skeleton and dense accumulation in right infradiaphragmatic region. This was confirmed at surgery as abscess. (A) anterior, (B) posterior, (C) right lateral, and (D) left lateral.

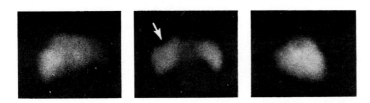

Fig. 19-8. Routine ^{99m}Tc-sulfur colloid liver study in patient of Fig. 19-7 showing corresponding defect (arrow). (Study courtesy of Robert E. O'Mara.)

tained from a ^{81}Rb generator. With its 190-keV monoenergetic photons it can be used to obtain high-resolution images of the cardiopulmonary and cerebral vascular system with a subsequent ventilation lung study (*12*). The low radiation dose and short half-life would permit serial studies when indicated (Fig. 19-6).

Adrenal Imaging

While pediatric endocrinology has been aided greatly by the in vitro procedures mentioned by Kaplan, the Michigan group has made remarkable progress in adrenal imaging (*13*). This may also prove a valuable clinical tool in the near future, but use in the pediatric age group may be limited by the high radiation dose.

Inflammatory Diseases

Of perhaps even greater clinical impact is the use of the agent ^{67}Ga-citrate (originally used for bone and tumor imaging) to detect sites of occult septic lesions (*14*). Figures 19-7 and 19-8 show the precise localization of a right subphrenic abscess in a 3-year-old boy with granulomatous disease of childhood and spiking fever using ^{67}Ga-citrate.

Summary

These brief thoughts, coupled with the innovative instrument and computer technological advances presented by Powell and Budinger and the almost daily development of new radiopharmaceuticals, make it clear that we are limited only by our imagination and diligence in the search for safer, faster, less traumatic, reproducible, and reliable studies with minimal radiation exposure. All of these are desirable indications for the application of nuclear medicine procedures in clinical pediatrics.

Acknowledgment

Renal studies shown in this chapter are from work supported in part by funds received from general research support Grants 5SOL RR 05470-08 from NIH.

References

1. DUSZYNSKI DO, JEWETT TC, ALLEN JE: Tc-99m Na pertechnetate scanning of the abdomen with particular reference to small bowel pathology. *Am J Roentgenol Radium Ther Nucl Med* 113: 258–262, 1971

2. KILPATRICK ZM, ASERON CA: Radioisotope detection of Meckel's diverticulum causing acute rectal hemorrhage. *N Engl J Med* 287: 653–654, 1972

3. BERQUIST TH, NOLAN NG, ADSON MA, et al: Diagnosis of Meckel's diverticulum by radioisotope scanning. *Mayo Clin Proc* 48: 98–102, 1973

4. LIN TH, KHENTIGAN A, WINCHELL HS: A ^{99m}Tc-labeled replacement for ^{131}I Rose Bengal in liver and biliary tract studies. *J Nucl Med* 15: 613–615, 1974

5. DUGAL P, EIKMAN EA, NATARAJAN TK, et al: A quantitative test of gallbladder function. *J Nucl Med* 13: 428, 1972

6. HANDMAKER H, McRAE J, BUCK EG: Intravenous radionuclide voiding cystography (IRVC)—an atraumatic method of demonstrating vesicoureteral reflux. *Radiology* 108: 703–705, 1973

7. LIN TH, KHENTIGAN A, WINCHELL HS: A ^{99m}Tc chelate substitute for organoradiomercurial renal agents. *J Nucl Med* 15: 34–35, 1974

8. DAVIES ER: Renal scintigraphy in pyelonephritis. *Proc R Soc Med* 64: 63–64, 1971

9. DAVIES ER: Topographical scintigraphy of the kidney. *Br Med Bull* 28: 205–209, 1972

10. HANDMAKER H, YOUNG BW, STUTZMAN ER: Clinical experience with ^{99m}Tc-DMSA (dimercaptosuccinic acid), a new renal imaging agent. *J Nucl Med* 15: 499, 1974

11. HANDMAKER H, PALMER DW, YOUNG BW: Simplified differential renal function studies using ^{99m}Tc-DMSA. Presented at RSNA, Dec 1974

12. YANO Y, McRAE J, ANGER HO: Lung function studies using short-lived ^{81m}Kr and the scintillation camera. *J Nucl Med* 11: 674–679, 1970

13. MOSES DC, BEIERWALTES WH: Adrenal imaging in children with ^{131}I-labeled cholesterol. *J Nucl Med* 14: 634, 1973

14. LITTENBERG RL, TAKETA RM, ALAZRAKI NP, et al: Gallium-67 for localization of septic lesions. *Ann Intern Med* 79: 403–406, 1973

Appendix

The rapidly changing field of nuclear medicine coupled with peculiarities imposed by pediatric patients (i.e., need for sedation, attention to dosimetry, etc.) have produced numerous problems to those individuals practicing, even on a limited basis, "pediatric nuclear medicine". The authors have attempted to provide an appendix containing data to aid these individuals. Included are:

Table A-1: The preferred sedation "cocktail" for pediatric patients when needed to perform imaging studies.

Tables A-2 and A-3: General schedule for calculation of pediatric radionuclide doses, based on surface area.

Table A-4A, B, and C: Suggested radionuclide doses for performance of the more common nuclear medicine procedures (developed empirically).

Table A-5A and B: Radiation doses to critical organ and gonads from the various procedures for various age groups.

Table A-6: Radiation dose from a variety of radiological procedures (for comparison to Table A-5).

Table A-7: Normal thyroid uptakes for a variety of ages.

Table A-8: Normal blood volume estimates for pediatric patients.

Table A-9: Normal sizes for a variety of organs imaged in nuclear medicine.

Fig. A-1: Size of kidney at various ages.

Sedation "Cocktail" for Imaging in Pediatric Patients

Children between the ages of 6 months and 3 years generally require sedation. Infants less than 6 months can usually be immobilized without difficulty. Older children who understand the purpose and importance of the procedure may not require sedation. For those children who do require sedation, Table A-1 gives the appropriate sedation mixture. This table was provided by J. J. Conway (reprinted from *Semin Nucl Med 2:* 305–315, 1972).

TABLE A-1. Sedation Mixture*

Meperidine hydrochloride (Demerol)	50 mg/cc
Promethazine hydrochloride (Phenergan)	25 mg/cc
Chlorpromazine (Thorazine)	25 mg/cc
Weight in pounds	**cc of each**
10–20	0.2
20–40	0.5
40–60	0.6
60–80	0.7
80–100	0.8
100+	1.0

Calculation of Pediatric Dose on Basis of Surface Area

Tables A-2 and A-3, provided by E. G. Bell, give the calculation of pediatric dose based on surface area with the patient's weight in pounds and kilograms. The metabolic activity is more accurately defined as a function of surface area than age, body height, or body weight. The surface area may be approximated by a power function of the body weight $(Bwt)^{0.7}$. The unity figure for the multiplier assumes a body weight of 65 kg or surface area of 1.7 m^2.

Example:

Body weight of infant = 6 kg (13.2 lb.)
Adult dose for bone scan = 15 mCi ^{99m}Tc-diphosphonate
Multiplier = 0.19
Infant dose = 15 × 0.19 = 3.0 mCi.

TABLE A-2. Schedule for Calculation of Pediatric Doses with Patient's Weight in Kilograms

Weight (kg)	Surface area (m^2)	Multiplier for adult dose
2	0.15	0.09
3	0.20	0.12
4	0.24	0.14
5	0.29	0.17
6	0.32	0.19
7	0.36	0.21
8	0.39	0.23
9	0.43	0.25
10	0.46	0.27
15	0.61	0.36
20	0.75	0.44
25	0.87	0.51
30	0.99	0.58
35	1.11	0.65
40	1.21	0.71
45	1.31	0.77
50	1.41	0.83
55	1.51	0.89
60	1.62	0.95
65	1.70	1.00

TABLE A-3. Schedule for Calculation of Pediatric Doses with Patient's Weight in Pounds

Weight (lb)	Surface area (m^2)	Multiplier for adult dose
5	0.17	0.10
10	0.27	0.16
15	0.36	0.21
20	0.43	0.25
25	0.51	0.30
30	0.58	0.34
40	0.70	0.41
50	0.82	0.48
60	0.92	0.54
70	1.04	0.61
80	1.14	0.67
90	1.22	0.72
100	1.33	0.78
110	1.41	0.83
120	1.50	0.88
130	1.60	0.94
140	1.68	0.99
143	1.70	1.00

Suggested Radionuclide Doses for Pediatric Procedures

The calculations and stated dose suggestions are to be guidelines for application by individuals in their own laboratories. Considerations of individual patient conditions, pathological processes, and physiology must be taken into account in determining the dose to be used in performing all nuclear medicine procedures in children. It is hoped that the figures in Tables A-4A, B, and C will be useful, but they reflect only the authors' opinion, based on our experience and that solicited from others in the field.

TABLE A-4A. Suggested Radionuclide Dose Schedules (General)

Weight (kg)	Brain (^{99m}TcO$_4^-$ * or ^{99m}Tc-DTPA) (mCi)	Kidney (^{99m}Tc-DTPA) (mCi)	Lung (^{99m}Tc-MAA) Liver (^{99m}Tc-SC) (mCi)	Liver (^{131}I-rose bengal)† (μCi)	Bone (^{99m}Tc-phosphate) (mCi)	Cister-nography (^{111}In-DTPA) (μCi)
1	2	1	0.40	25	2	50
2	2	1	0.40	25	2	50
3	2	1	0.40	25	2	50
4	2	1	0.40	25	2	50
5	2	1	0.40	25	3	50
6	2	1	0.40	25	3	50
7	2	1	0.40	25	3	50
8	2	1	0.40	25	3	50
9	2	1	0.40	25	3	50
10	2	1	0.40	25	4	50
11	2.2	1.1	0.44	50	4	50
12	2.4	1.2	0.44	50	4	50
13	2.6	1.3	0.52	50	4	52
14	2.8	1.4	0.56	50	4	56
15	3.0	1.5	0.60	50	4	60
16	3.2	1.6	0.64	50	4	64
17	3.4	1.7	0.68	50	4	68
18	3.6	1.8	0.72	50	4	72
19	3.8	1.9	0.76	50	4	76
20	4.0	2.0	0.80	50	5	80
21	4.2	2.1	0.84	50	5	84
22	4.4	2.2	0.88	50	5	88
23	4.6	2.3	0.92	50	5	92
24	4.8	2.4	0.96	50	5	96
25	5.0	2.5	1.00	50	5	100
26	5.2	2.6	1.04	50	5	104
27	5.4	2.7	1.08	50	5	108
28	5.6	2.8	1.12	50	5	112
29	5.8	2.9	1.16	50	5	116
30	6.0	3.0	1.20	50	5	120
31	6.2	3.1	1.24	50	5.2	124
32	6.4	3.2	1.28	50	5.4	128
33	6.6	3.3	1.32	50	5.6	132
34	6.8	3.4	1.36	50	5.8	136
35	7.0	3.5	1.40	50	6.0	140

Weight (kg)	Brain (^{99m}TcO$_4^-$ * or ^{99m}Tc-DTPA) (mCi)	Kidney (^{99m}Tc-DTPA) (mCi)	Lung (^{99m}Tc-MAA) Liver (^{99m}Tc-SC) (mCi)	Liver (^{131}I-rose bengal)† (μCi)	Bone (^{99m}Tc-phosphate) (mCi)	Cister-nography (^{111}In-DTPA) (μCi)
36	7.2	3.6	1.44	50	6.2	144
37	7.4	3.7	1.48	50	6.4	148
38	7.6	3.8	1.52	50	6.6	152
39	7.8	3.9	1.56	50	6.8	156
40	8.0	4.0	1.60	100	7.0	160
41	8.2	4.1	1.64	100	7.2	164
42	8.4	4.2	1.68	100	7.4	168
43	8.6	4.3	1.72	100	7.6	172
44	8.8	4.4	1.76	100	7.8	176
45	9.0	4.5	1.80	100	8.0	180
46	9.2	4.6	1.84	100	8.2	184
47	9.4	4.7	1.88	100	8.4	188
48	9.6	4.8	1.92	100	8.6	192
49	9.8	4.9	1.96	100	8.8	196
50	10.0	5.0	2.00	100	9.0	200
51	10.2	5.0	2.04	100	9.2	204
52	10.4	5.0	2.08	100	9.4	208
53	10.6	5.0	2.12	100	9.6	212
54	10.8	5.0	2.16	100	9.8	216
55	11.0	5.0	2.20	100	10.0	220
56	11.2	5.0	2.24	100	10.2	224
57	11.4	5.0	2.28	100	10.4	228
58	11.6	5.0	2.32	100	10.6	232
59	11.8	5.0	2.36	100	10.8	236
60	12.0	5.0	2.40	150	11.0	240

* If ^{99m}Tc used as pertechnetate, block thyroid uptake with KClO$_4$, 8–15 mg/kg.
† Block thyroid with Lugol's solution before injection and on subsequent days when indicated.
Table provided by H. Handmaker.

TABLE A-4B. Suggested Radionuclide Dose Schedule (Thyroid Studies)

Test	Radionuclide	Dose (μCi)
Thyroid uptake	^{123}I	100
	^{125}I	50
Thyroid scan or scintiphoto*	^{123}I	100
$_3$ (Cytomel) suppression test	Following uptake, place on Cytomel 3μg/kg/24 hr for 7 days and repeat uptake, correcting for background.	

* Imaging performed 3 hr after ingestion of capsule.
Table provided by H. Handmaker.

Test	Radionuclide	Dose (μCi/kg)
Platelet survival studies	^{51}Cr	4.3
Ferrokinetics	^{59}Fe-citrate	0.14
Schilling test	^{57}Co-B_{12}	0.007
Bone marrow imaging	^{52}Fe	1.4
	^{111}InCl$_3$	30
	^{99m}Tc-sulfur colloid	86
Plasma volume	^{125}I-IHSA	0.07
	^{99m}Tc-albumin	4.3
	^{113m}In-transferrin	14.3
Red blood cell mass	^{51}Cr-labeled RBC	0.43
	^{99m}Tc-Sn-RBC	4.3
Red blood cell survival	^{51}Cr-labeled RBC	1.4

Table provided by D. C. Price and C. Ries.

Radiation Dose from Pediatric Nuclear Medicine Procedures

Table A-5A on the next two pages gives the estimated radiation dose in millirads per microcurie administered to various organs from different nuclear medicine procedures. Table A-5B (page 277) gives the total-body dose for various blood volume procedures. Both tables were provided by E. L. Saenger and J. G. Kereiakes.

TABLE A-5A. Radiation Dose (mrad/μCi Administered) to Critical Organ and Gonad for Selected Radiopharmaceuticals

Scintigraphic study	Agent	Avg. admin. dose	Organ	Radiation dose by age of patients					
				Newborn	1 yr	5 yr	10 yr	15 yr	Standard man
Brain	^{99m}Tc (pertechnetate)	200 μCi/kg	Gut	1.60	0.40	0.30	0.20	0.13	0.10
			Gonads						
			M	0.102	0.079	0.073	0.066	0.014	0.012
			F	0.219	0.076	0.045	0.032	0.022	0.018
Thyroid	^{123}I	100 μCi/kg	Thyroid	160	109	51	30	21	15
			Gonads						
			M	0.085	0.066	0.061	0.055	0.012	0.010
			F	0.244	0.084	0.050	0.036	0.024	0.020
Lung	^{99m}Tc-macroaggregated albumin	40 μCi/kg	Lung	1.83	0.65	0.40	0.24	0.19	0.14
			Gonads						
			M	0.060	0.046	0.043	0.038	0.008	0.007
			F	0.110	0.038	0.022	0.016	0.010	0.009
Liver	^{99m}Tc-sulfur colloid	40 μCi/kg	Liver	2.3	1.1	0.6	0.4	0.3	0.3
			Gonads						
			M	0.161	0.125	0.116	0.104	0.023	0.019
			F	0.280	0.097	0.058	0.041	0.028	0.023

(Continued)

TABLE 5A. Continued

Scintigraphic study	Agent	Avg. admin. dose	Organ	Radiation dose by age of patients					
				Newborn	1 yr	5 yr	10 yr	15 yr	Standard man
Kidney	^{99m}Tc-DTPA	100 μCi/kg	Bladder	4.9	1.8	1.2	0.8	0.6	0.5
			Gonads						
			M	0.170	0.132	0.122	0.110	0.024	0.020
			F	0.329	0.113	0.068	0.049	0.032	0.027
Bone	^{99m}Tc-phosphates	Approx. 150 μCi/kg	Bladder (void 1 hr)	0.90	0.29	0.17	0.11	0.09	0.07
			Bladder (no void)	6.27	2.06	1.19	0.76	0.58	0.49
			Skeleton	1.50	0.52	0.20	0.11	0.064	0.045
			Gonads						
			M	0.289	0.224	0.207	0.187	0.041	0.034
			F	0.561	0.193	0.115	0.083	0.055	0.046
Cardiac	^{99m}Tc-albumin	Approx. 125 μCi/kg	Whole body	0.20	0.07	0.04	0.03	0.023	0.02
			Gonads						
			M	0.340	0.264	0.244	0.220	0.048	0.040
			F	0.658	0.227	0.135	0.097	0.065	0.054
Blood volume	^{125}I-IHSA	5—20 μCi/kg depending on weight	Whole body	14.40	4.10	1.54	1.03	0.68	0.60
			Gonads						
			M	6.40	4.38	2.04	1.20	0.86	0.60
			F	9.50	3.28	1.95	1.41	0.93	0.78

TABLE A-5B. Whole-Body Doses (mrads/μCi Administered) from Blood-Volume Measurements*

Agent	Whole-body dose by age					Standard man
	Newborn	1 yr	5 yr	10 yr	15 yr	
^{125}I-albumin	14.40	4.10	1.54	1.03	0.68	0.60
^{131}I-albumin	32.0	10.0	6.0	4.0	2.4	2.0
^{99m}Tc-albumin	0.20	0.07	0.04	0.03	0.023	0.02
^{51}Cr-red blood cells	7.0	2.5	1.5	1.0	0.6	0.5
^{99m}Tc-red blood cells	0.20	0.07	0.04	0.03	0.023	0.02

* Adapted from Ball and Wolf (Chapter 16, Ref. *44*).

Average Radiation Exposure for Radiographic Procedures

Table A-6, provided by H. Handmaker, shows the radiation doses from selected radiologic procedures for comparison with equivalent nuclear medicine procedures.

TABLE A-6. Average Radiation Exposure for Radiographic Procedures (mrads)

Procedure	Organ	Exposure at age (yr)				
		Under 2	2–4	5–9	10–14	Adult*
Voiding urethrocystography† with 70 mm fluorography	Gonads					
	Male	305	79	63	43	
	Female	—	255	270	299	
Chest (PA)‡	Gonads					
	Male					0.02
	Female					0.04
Abdomen (AP)‡	Gonads					
	Male					12 (7)‖
	Female					51
Intravenous urogram‡	Gonads					
	Male					60 (18)‖
	Female					132

* Pediatric exposures not available.
† Kaude J V, Lorenz E, Reed J M: Gonad dose to children in voiding urethrocystography performed with 70-mm image-intensifier fluorography. *Radiology* 92: 771–774, 1969.
‡ Antoku S, Russell W J: Dose to the active bone marrow, gonads, and skin from roentgenography and fluoroscopy. *Radiology* 101: 669–678, 1971.
‖ Lead protector.

Radioiodine Uptake Values for Different Age Groups

Table A-7, provided by D. A. Fisher, gives the radioiodine uptake values for different age groups. Values given are for 300 μg/day iodine intake, with bracketed values based on 700 μg/day intake for euthyroid subjects without goiter. Data are for oral radioiodine administration and exclude thigh correction. In patients with goiter, uptake values average 0.85–0.90 of the listed results. The data were generated by computer. Programming was based on absolute uptake measurements conducted in various areas of the United States to determine the influence of age and iodine intake on thyroidal radioiodine uptake. Individual laboratories should establish normal values for their equipment and geographic area.

TABLE A-7. Radioiodine Uptake Values (%) for Different Age Groups* (90 Percentile Range)

Age (yr)	Uptake at various times		
	4 hr	6 hr	24 hr
5	9–31 (6–21)	8–36 (6–25)	10–43 (6–31)
10	7–27 (5–19)	7–33 (5–23)	9–40 (6–30)
15	5–25 (4–17)	6–30 (4–21)	8–38 (5–29)
20–80	5–23 (4–17)	5–27 (4–20)	8–38 (6–30)

Estimated Blood Volumes

Table A-8 gives estimated blood volumes at various ages. This table was provided by D. C. Price and C. Ries.

TABLE A-8. Estimated Blood Volumes

Age	Plasma volume (cc/kg) (PV)	Red cell mass (cc/kg) (RCM)	Total blood volume (cc/kg)		References
			(from PV)	(from RCM)	
Newborn	41.3	43.1	82.1	86.1	1
	46			84.7	2
			78		6
1–7 days	51–54		82–86		6
		37.9		77.8	5
1–12 mo	46.1		78.1		4
		25.5		72.8	5
1–3 yr	44.4		73.8		3
	47.2		81.8		4
		24.9		69.1	5
4–6 yr	48.5		80.0		3
	49.6		85.6		4
		25.5		67.5	5
7–9 yr	52.2		87.6		3
	49.0		86.1		4
		24.3		67.5	5
10–12 yr	51.9		87.6		3
	46.2		83.2		4
		26.3		67.4	5
13–15 yr	51.2		88.3		3
16–18 yr	50.1		90.2		3
Adults	39–44	25–30	68–88	55–75	7

References:

1. Jegier W, MacLaurin J, Blankenship W, et al: Comparative study of blood volume estimation in the newborn infant using I^{131}-labeled human serum albumin (IHSA) and T-1824. *Scand J Clin Lab Invest* 16: 125–132, 1964

2. Mollison P L, Veall N, Cutbush M: Red cell and plasma volume in newborn infants. *Arch Dis Child* 25: 242–253, 1950

3. Morse M, Cassels D E, Schlutz F W: Blood volume of normal children. *Am J Physiol* 151: 448–458, 1947

4. Russell S J M: Blood volume studies in healthy children. *Arch Dis Child* 24: 88–98, 1949

5. Sukarochana K, Parenzan L, Thakurdas N, et al: Red cell mass determinations in infancy and childhood, with the use of radioactive chromium. *J Pediatr* 59: 903–908, 1961

6. Usher R, Shephard M, Lind J: The blood volume of the newborn infant and placental transfusion. *Acta Paediatr Scand* 52: 497–512, 1963

7. Wagner H N, ed: *Principles of Nuclear Medicine*, Philadelphia, W B Saunders, 1968, pp 838–841

Body Weights and Organ Weights

Table A-9, given on the next page, shows the weight in grams of various organs during growth. This table was provided by E. L. Saenger and J. C. Kereiakes.

TABLE A-9. Body Weights and Organ Weights (gm) for Various Ages

Organ	Weights in grams at age					
	Newborn	1 yr	5 yr	10 yr	15 yr	Standard man
Whole body	3,540	12,100	20,300	33,500	55,000	70,000
Brain	350	945	1,241	1,313	1,350	1,400
Heart	20	47	86	140	209	298
Intestines	146	398	550	820	1,350	1,700
Kidneys	23	72	112	187	247	300
Liver	136	333	591	918	1,289	1,700
Lungs	52	172	291	523	701	1,000
Pancreas	2.8	14	23	30	68	80
Spleen	9.4	31	54	101	138	150
Stomach	6.5	27	57	90	120	160
Thyroid	1.9 (1.5)*	2.5 (2.2)	6.1 (4.7)	8.7 (8.0)	15.8 (11.2)	20 (16)
Testes	0.67	1.5	1.7	2.0	18	28
Ovaries	0.29	1.0	2.0	3.5	6.5	8.5

* Thyroid weights in parentheses are from the recent data of Wellman H, Kereiakes J, Bramson B: Total and partial-body counting of children for radiopharmaceutical dosimetry data. In Medical Radionuclides: Radiation Dose and Effects. Cloutier R J, Edwards C L, Snyder W S, eds. Symposium Series 20, CONF-691212. Oak Ridge, Tenn. USAEC, TID, 1970, pp 133—156.
Table provided by E. L. Saenger and J. C. Kereiakes.

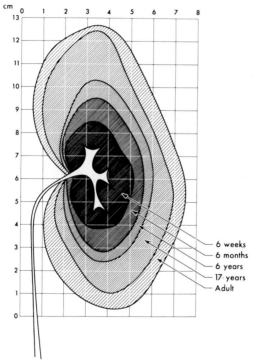

Fig. A-1. Size of kidney at various ages. Stylized renal growth diagram (based on measurements from random series using urographic techniques). Courtesy of Bradford W. Young.

Index

Hematoma, see *Brain*
Hemoglobin A, 181
Hemorrhage, subarachnoid, 30
Hepatitis, 92, 95, 98, 111, 262
Histogram, 86–88, 247
Hodgkin's disease, 108, 149
Hologram, 232
Hormones
    FSH, LH, sex steroids, radioim-
        munoassay, 196–199
    human growth, radioimmunoassay,
        193–195
    progesterone   radioimmunoassay,
        199
    thyroid production, 46, 47
Howell-Jolly bodies, 114–115
Hyaline membrane disease, 60–62, 67
Hydrocephalus
    brain scan, 10, 12
    communicating, 26, 28–35, 38–40
    compensation, 30–31
    noncommunicating, 30–32, 34
Hydrogen-3
    -digoxin, 188
    -glycosides, 188
    -hormone, radioimmunoassay, 193
Hypothalamic-leutenizing factor, 198
Hypothalamus, 17, 196–199

I

Image display, see *Display*
Impulse response, 253–254
Indium, 134
Indium-111, bleomycin, 152–153, 156
Indium-111, chloride
    bone marrow imaging, 173, 273
    brain studies, 14
    transferrin binding, 153
    tumor staging, 152–153
Indium-111, DTPA, 24, 38, 272
Indium-113m
    -chloride, 13, 14
    colloid, spleen imaging, 105
    equilibrium dose constants, 222
    lung agent, 60
    -transferrin, 158, 159, 273
Infarct, see *Brain, Heart*
Infection
    abscess, 7, 16, 92, 93, 111–112, 153,
        206–207, 265, 266
    aspergillus niger, 153
    encephalitis, 17
    intracranial, 37–38
    peripheral extension of bone mar-
        row, 175
    pneumonia, 63–64, 67

spleen, 110–112
    viral bronchiolitis, 65, 67
Injection
    cardiovascular shunt, 82–83, 85–86
    cisternography techniques, 24–26,
        35, 36, 41
    vs. oral dose, thyroid uptake, 49
Instrumentation, 231–241
    see also *specific instrument*
    angiocardiography, 69–70, 83, 250
    bone marrow imaging, 173–174
    bone scanning, 137–138
    cardiovascular shunt quantitation,
        83
    cisternography, 26
    kidney imaging, 120–121, 239, 244
    lung imaging, 60
    renogram, 119, 120
    thyroid uptake, 49; imaging, 52
Insulin, 194, 195
Intestines, see *Gastrointestinal tract*
Intravenous pyelogram, 158, 276
Iodine-123
    equilibrium dose constants, 222
    nuclear parameters, 3, 48
    thyroid studies, 218, 219, 224, 225,
        273, 274
Iodine-125
    -digoxigenin, 188
    equilibrium dose constants, 222
    -HSA, blood volume, 273, 275, 276
    -HSA, plasma volume, 159–160
    -HSA, radiation dosimetry, 158, 159
    nuclear parameters, 46, 48
    thyroid, 219, 223, 224, 273
Iodine-131
    cyclotron production, 2, 3
    -diodrast, 84
    equilibrium dose constants, 222
    -hormones, radioimmunoassay, 193
    lung agents, 60
    nuclear parameters, 46, 48
    thyroid, 55, 150–151, 218, 219, 223,
        224
Iodine-131, albumin
    cisternography, 24
    plasma volume, 159
    radiation dose, 157–159, 220, 223,
        224, 226
    uptake by cyst, hygroma, 32–33
Iodine-131, Hippuran, 119–120, 126–
    128, 131
Iodine-131, rose bengal
    clearance, 90–91, 92, 97–99
    liver imaging, 89, 90, 223, 272
    radiation dosimetry, 99, 220, 223
    spleen uptake, 115
Iodine-131, triolein, 220

lesion detectability, 92
motion artifact, 92, 96–97, 248, 253, 257
portal hypertension, 111
platelet survival, 164, 165, 166
radiation dose, 106, 221, 223, 274
radionuclide
  ^{198}Au-colloid, 89
  ^{131}I-rose bengal, 89, 90
  ^{99m}Mo-molybdate, 89
  ^{99m}Tc-mercaptocarboxylate, 262
  ^{99m}Tc-sulfur colloid, 89, 90
subtraction, pancreas imaging, 252
-to-spleen activity ratio, 107, 164–166
trauma, laceration, 93
tumor, 94–96, 153, 154
weight, 217, 222, 278
Lugol's, 24, 99, 224
Lung, 57–67, 71–74, 81–88, 204
angiocardiogram, 71–74, 264
cardiovascular shunt quantitation, 81–88
development, 57–58
disorders
  bacterial pneumonia, 63
  bronchial asthma, 67
  bronchiolitis, 65
  bronchopulmonary sequestration, 67
  congenital emphysema, 67
  congenital lobar emphysema, 62
  cystic fibrosis, 66 & 67
  foreign body aspiration, 67
  pulmonary agenesis, 67
  pulmonary emboli, 67
  pulmonary vascular occlusion, 65
  spontaneous pulmonary vascular occlusive disease, 67
dose, ^{99m}Tc-MAA, 272
fetal and postnatal development, 57
foreign bodies, 62–64, 67
hyaline membrane disease, 60–62, 67
instrumentation, 60
mediastinal lesion, 153
metastatic disease, 150, 151, 153
motion correction, 253
perfusion, regional, 58–59, 254
radiation dose, 223, 274, 276
radionuclides
  ^{113m}In or ^{131}I particles, 60
  ^{99m}Tc-macroaggregate, 58
  ^{99m}Tc-microspheres, 60
  ^{125}Xe, 60
  ^{133}Xe, 59
thrombosis, 65–67
transmission imaging, 93

tuberculosis, 15, 16
ventilation, 59–60, 254, 257
volume, 59, 60
weight, 217, 278
Lutetium, 134
Lymph nodes
see also Hodgkin's disease
^{198}Au imaging, 149
Lymphoma, 108, 152

M

Magnesium, 134
Malaria, 110, 111
Matrix
  Anger camera, 244, 246
  computer, 239, 244–245
  whole-body scanner, 244
Meckel's diverticulum, 204, 208, 261
Mediastinal lesion, 153
Meningitis, 10, 15, 16, 30, 37–38, 206–207
Mercury-197
  kidney imaging, 120
  equilibrium dose constants, 222
  -chlormerodrin, 221, 223
Mercury-203
  equilibrium dose constants, 222
  -chlormerodrin, 120, 223
MIRD absorbed-dose calculation, 213–216
Molybdenum-99, molybdate, 89
Motion artifact, 92, 96–97, 253, 257
MTF, Anger camera, 246
Multi-wire proportional chamber, 236–238, 246
Muscle, 221
Myeloid metaplasia, 170

N

Neonatal, see *Newborn*
Neohydrin, see chlormerodrin
Neutron activation analysis, 181–182
Newborn
  cumulative thyroid uptake, 218
  field of view, 241, 247
  hepatitis, 95, 98, 262
  lung development, 57–58
  pinhole collimator imaging, 241
  radiation dose, 158, 223
  renal masses, 127
  serum digoxin level, 189–190
  suggested radiation dose limits, 216
  thyroid uptake, 49, 216
  weight, body and organ, 217, 222
Niemann-Pick reticulosis, 113

X

Xenon
  gas, pressurized MWPC, 236–238
  liquid, detector, 238, 240
Xenon-125, 60
Xenon-133
  equilibrium dose constants, 222
  myocardial blood flow, 254
  lung perfusion, 59, 62, 63, 66, 67
  lung ventilation, 59–61, 65, 66
X-ray
  compared to bone imaging, 133,
    140–144, 146, 204, 225
  contrast angiocardiograms, 81
  lung, 150, 151
  radiation dose, 276
x-y position, see *Resolution, spatial*

Y

Yttrium, 134

Z

Zirconium, 134